Effectiveness of interventions to promote healthy eating in elderly people living in the community: a review

HEALTH EDUCATION AUTHORITY

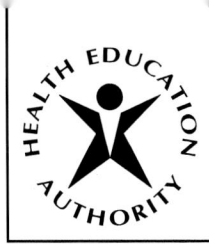

Effectiveness of interventions to promote healthy eating in elderly people living in the community: a review

Astrid Fletcher
Christine Rake

**Department of Epidemiology and
Population Health
London School of Hygiene and
Tropical Medicine**

HEA Project Team

Jane Meyrick   Research Project Manager
Antony Morgan   Head of Monitoring and Effectiveness Research

---

In the same series:

Health promotion in older people for the prevention of coronary heart disease and stroke

Health promotion in childhood and young adolescence for the prevention of unintentional injuries

Effectiveness of video for health education

Effectiveness of mental health promotion interventions

Health promotion with young people for the prevention of substance misuse

Health promotion interventions to promote healthy eating in the general population

Effectiveness of oral health promotion

Effectiveness of interventions to promote healthy feeding of infants under one year: a review

Effectiveness of interventions to promote healthy eating in preschool children aged 1–5 years: a review

Effectiveness of interventions to promote healthier living in people from minority ethnic groups: a review

Effectiveness of interventions to promote healthy eating in pregnant women and women of childbearing age: a review

Forthcoming topics:

Health promotion interventions in the workplace: a review

© Health Education Authority, 1998

ISBN 0 7521 1094 2

Health Education Authority
Trevelyan House
30 Great Peter Street
London SW1P 2HW

Designed by Edwin Belchamber
Typeset by Wayzgoose
Cover design by Mario Grasso
Printed in Great Britain

Contents

Acknowledgements
The authors would like to thank Sue Prior (Epidemiology Unit, Epidemiology and Population Health, London School of Hygiene and Tropical Medicine) and Professor Prakash Shetty (Human Nutrition Unit, Epidemiology and Population Health, London School of Hygiene and Tropical Medicine) for their help and advice during the course of this review. This study was funded by the Health Education Authority.

Structure of the report

This report is divided into three main sections: the executive summary, the main report and appendices.

The executive summary summarises the main findings and recommendations of the report. The main report contains the background information, methodology, scope of review and definitions used (Chapter 1). This is followed by the detailed findings of all the studies reviewed and general overview of these results (Chapters 2 and 3), and a few studies in the general population with some breakdown by age (Chapter 4). The main report also contains descriptions of some key demonstration studies (but which lack a full evaluation) and new initiatives and a brief view of current work being undertaken in the United Kingdom (Chapter 5). The conclusions and recommendations are presented (Chapter 6). Finally, the appendices detail the literature search methodology and results, summary tables of studies reviewed, the data extraction form and the individuals and organisations contacted.

Studies in the present review are identified by the name(s) of the authors and the date of publication.

Target audience
The review is intended for policy specialists in nutrition and public health, health educationalists, and those concerned with health promotion, practising dietitians and health visitors working with elderly people and academic researchers with an interest in the nutrition of elderly people.

Preface

The Health Education Authority (HEA) welcomes this new review of effectiveness of healthy eating interventions in elderly people living in the community as one means of gathering evidence for health promotion. It forms one of an HEA series of systematic reviews that have begun to address the need for an evidence base in Health Promotion. This report provides an exhaustive review of the available evidence and highlights the importance for health promoters to not only evaluate their work but to evaluate it well in order to increase the body of work reviews can draw on.

This report is one in a set of linked reviews within the HEA series of effectiveness reviews of health promotion interventions which examine healthy eating in various populations. The need to focus on these populations was identified in an earlier review in the HEA series examining healthy eating in the general population[1] but is also in response to the findings of previous reviews that health promotion work is more effective if targeted at specific population groups.

This report is published alongside a set of sister reviews, of 'Opportunities for and barriers to change' in the same target groups, commissioned by the Department of Health[2] to examine the behavioural patterns, attitudes and cultural values which might provide opportunities for, or constitute barriers to, healthy eating. The two sets of reviews are complementary in their scope and coverage of the literature and while individual studies may appear in more than one review, they are covered from different perspectives.

The aim of systematic reviews

The commitment within the NHS to move towards evidence-based practice has, to some extent, been mirrored within health promotion. For this reason the methodological tool used to find evidence, the systematic review, has been applied to a range of health promotion topics in an effort to inform health professionals in addition to increasing the knowledge base about effective health promotion.

---

[1]Roe *et al.* (1997) *Health promotion interventions to promote healthy eating in the general population: a review*. London: Health Education Authority.

[2]*Opportunities for, and barriers to, change in dietary behaviour in elderly people.* (To be published summer 1998).

Executive summary

The growing number of elderly people in the United Kingdom highlight the need to identify interventions and strategies to maintain and enhance their health. This report reviews the studies of interventions to promote healthy eating in elderly people living in the community. Interventions in settings such as long-stay care or provision of meals programmes were not included. The definition of healthy eating in elderly people includes maintenance of adequate nutrition and prevention of nutritional deficiencies as well as a diet to reduce disease risk, primarily cardiovascular (CVD) risk.

Main findings

Lack of good quality studies

Our search revealed a large literature on nutrition interventions in the elderly and a paucity of evaluative studies. Most of these studies were of poor quality. The overwhelming impression from the literature is an enthusiastic endorsement for interventions to promote healthy eating in elderly people. This is not supported by our review.

We identified only 23 studies which met our criteria and which included some description of the nutrition intervention and nutrition outcomes. We accepted some study designs that would not be capable of providing good scientific evidence because we wanted to provide a comprehensive picture of the range and quality of such 'evaluative' studies that have been undertaken.

Of the 23 studies, only eight used a randomised control design while eight were non-randomised controlled experimental studies, and seven were uncontrolled studies. Twenty-one of the 23 studies were carried out in the US, one in Australia and one in France. There were no studies from the UK.

The most common studies were studies of nutrition interventions undertaken in the setting of an elderly community programme (18 studies). Many of these studies had serious methodological faults. Most commonly they were: small and underpowered; used a non-random control group or were uncontrolled; and relied on self-reported data, mostly with no attention to validity of outcome measures. A few studies had high withdrawal rates or missing data and many used inappropriate statistical analyses. None of the seven studies that used cluster allocation or randomisation employed the appropriate method of analysis.

Many small studies were conducted by single or dual authors suggesting limited resources had been committed to the studies. The generally well conducted studies were of multifactorial interventions in the context of adding health promotion to insurance policies (five studies). These were large, long-term, high resource studies conducted in the US.

Intervention strategy

Most studies used nutritional interventions to reduce CVD risk with an emphasis on low fat intakes, reduced salt and increased fruit and vegetables. Six studies used strategies to correct nutritional deficiencies in elderly people while two other studies appeared to combine both approaches. The strategy of the intervention was unclear in three others.

Evidence of effectiveness

Our review provided limited evidence for the effectiveness of healthy eating interventions in elderly people.

Two large positive trials which included nutrition as part of general health promotion showed some benefits, but the setting of the intervention in the context of the US health insurance scheme limits the applicability to the UK. These studies used interventions promoting healthy eating behaviours to reduce CVD risk (especially lower fat intake).

Two small studies in the setting of community programmes for elderly people also showed benefits; one of these studies specifically targeted elderly people at high risk of nutritional deficiencies while the other study used a multifactorial CHD risk approach.

None of these four studies had objective measures of outcome, and relied on self-reported dietary behaviour.

A strategy of individual feedback and goal setting tended to be associated with a positive intervention. There was some weak evidence for a benefit of small group programmes which also included social and physical activities.

There was a wide age range of elderly people but most studies did not have the power to examine differential effects of interventions with age. No studies considered the appropriateness of nutrition interventions according to age.

We found only a handful of studies that examined either policy or strategies directed at elderly people in the community. Even when elderly people were included in interventions directed at the whole community, no separate information on this age group was provided.

Most studies were conducted in the US where healthy eating awareness is higher than in the UK and has been promoted over two decades. This may further limit the generalisability of the studies to elderly people in the UK.

Summary of findings by setting

Nutrition interventions in elderly people in the community meal setting

Out of three published studies evaluating the effectiveness of a nutrition education programme in the context of community meal settings, only one study provided controlled and unconfounded evidence of the short-term benefits of the programme. Although response bias cannot be entirely discounted in this study, the large improvements in nutrition can be attributed in part to the programme. The success of the intervention is likely to be related to: (i) the focus on high-risk individuals with nutritionally inadequate diets; (ii) the use of a motivational group-led model; (iii) the emphasis on improving vitamin, protein and mineral intakes. The results are likely to be generalisable to similar settings with individuals at high risk of nutritional deficiencies but longer-term benefits and cost-effectiveness need to be demonstrated.

Nutrition interventions in elderly people in communal settings

None of the nine studies conducted in the setting of community programmes or housing projects for the elderly provides adequate evidence for a benefit of intervention although conversely none of them provides adequate evidence for no benefit. Only three studies were randomised controlled trials; two of these demonstrating a benefit of intervention used the weaker outcomes of self-reported dietary behaviours. One study showed quite impressive and favourable changes in cholesterol and HDL cholesterol compatible with the self-reported dietary changes but was not randomised and confounding and biased allocation may have occurred.

Taken together the studies provide weak evidence for improved eating behaviours in elderly people soon after nutrition or multifactorial interventions. Participants were mostly women but a range of income groups was represented across the studies. Most studies used the format of group-led activities which are less resource intensive than individual counselling.

Nutrition interventions in the elderly population living in the community

Evidence for the effect of nutrition interventions targeting elderly people in the general community is poor. There are no randomised controlled trials in this group of studies and only two controlled studies. The most promising result was from a study using a community strategy and focusing on promotion of wholemeal bread/wholegrains. This study took place in a small community and may not be feasible in larger population settings; it is likely that the intervention was resource intensive. Garden boxes and gardening and nutrition classes were the intervention strategy in an uncontrolled study with weak evidence of benefit from the programme. However, the strategy was an innovative one and deserves more rigorous evaluation.

Nutrition interventions as part of health promotion interventions

The studies of nutrition interventions in the context of health promotion were generally well designed and of adequate size to detect important differences in nutrition outcomes (though with some exceptions as noted above).

Although the concept of including nutrition as part of a general package of health promotion is attractive there are a variety of problems which limit the findings from these studies: (i) a range of preventive strategies was included in a single package and it is difficult, therefore, to attribute benefits (if any) to any particular component of the package; (ii) the nutrition content of the intervention was poorly described; (iii) inadequate process data were presented for the nutrition component.

Moreover, while health promotion is clearly an important strategy for public health, the marketing of health promotion programmes also offers the potential for considerable financial gains. A series of studies was financed by a major private insurance provider using a health promotion package in which the authors had a financial interest.

Several important trials of health promotion in elderly people had to be excluded from the review as there was no description of the nutrition intervention or nutrition outcomes.

Of the three randomised controlled trials with data available from a control group, only one study (the Bank of America Study) found benefits across a wide range of healthy eating habits promoted by the intervention. The study used a six-monthly computerised feedback to a lifestyle questionnaire. The San Diego study used face-to-face counselling and goal setting but the restriction to only one goal limited the opportunity for a dietary benefit although a small reduction in dietary fat was found. The Rural Health Promotion Project adopted a pragmatic approach to cholesterol counselling which was not successful in changing cholesterol levels.

In summary, the evidence suggests that a feedback/goal setting type intervention may lead to improved eating behaviours in elderly people but validation of self-reported changes is essential before uncritically accepting the benefits of such an approach.

Recommendations

Healthy eating interventions specifically targeting elderly people need further evaluation in the UK context. These interventions should implement nutritional guidelines for this age group and include minimum nutritional requirements for elderly people as well as interventions to reduce disease risk. It is likely that interventions using group participation with goal setting offer the best way of delivering the interventions.

The elderly are a heterogeneous group and more research is required to identify and evaluate healthy eating interventions in different age groups, gender, living and socioeconomic circumstances, and by health status.

Elderly people include those with nutritional deficiencies and those at risk of nutritional deficiencies, as well as those with adequate diets. Interventions promoting low fat, low calorie diets and weight reduction may be undesirable in some elderly people. Assessing individual dietary intake before promoting the appropriate nutritional intervention is an area which requires more attention.

Healthy eating interventions must therefore take account of differing nutritional requirements according to age and health status. Individual dietary assessment or a screening checklist requires further exploration.

Evaluation of healthy eating interventions in elderly people requires high quality randomised controlled studies using validated measures of outcome and including both objective and subjective measures of nutrient intake, and dietary behaviour.

More attention should be paid to methods for assessing nutritional status of elderly people, for example measurement of energy expenditure.

Innovative interventions, such as gardening projects and social programmes including physical activities, require further evaluation in view of their potential to enhance quality of life.

Nutritional interventions in elderly people may differ from those in middle age and younger populations. Dietary guidelines which more specifically address the prevention of disease and disability in populations are derived from longitudinal studies which to date have been conducted primarily in middle-aged people. There is far less evidence to inform nutritional recommendations for elderly people, in particular very elderly people. The acceptance and endorsement of healthy eating guidelines for elderly people by public health practitioners requires a stronger body of scientific evidence.

Healthy eating guidelines for elderly people should be based on appropriate evidence from epidemiological studies in elderly people on the associations between dietary intakes and disease risk. These data are particularly lacking in very elderly people.

1. Introduction

Background

The present review was commissioned by the Health Education Authority in parallel with a series of related reviews on the effectiveness of interventions to promote healthy eating in various populations. The focus of the current review is on interventions to promote healthy eating among elderly people.

The demographic perspective

Changes in fertility and mortality patterns have led to an increasing number of elderly people in the population of the UK. People aged over 65 years currently account for 18% of the population and this proportion is forecast to rise to 23% by 2030; an increase from 11 million to 14 million (Office for National Statistics, 1996). Of particular demographic importance are the predicted increases in the oldest old (over 75 years) from 6.8% to 10.7% and the high proportion of women relative to men in the elderly population. Many elderly women are widows and live alone (over 50% of women aged over 80) while elderly men are more likely to be cared for by their families (Department of Health, 1992a). Differences between rural and urban areas in these demographic trends are also observed. In general, cities have 'aged' more than other areas of the country.

Although the proportion of elderly people who are home owners and receive occupational and state pensions has increased, the average income of elderly people is considerably lower than the rest of the adult population. Elderly people living alone account for over 80% of the lowest single household income groups. Older women are of particular interest. The fact that the majority are widows and of lower socioeconomic status, compared both with men, and with younger ages, would appear to render them at a special disadvantage.

The imperatives for public health as a consequence of the aging of the population include: the need to identify strategies and interventions to improve the health and wellbeing of elderly people; the need to provide and deliver health care to elderly people.

Opportunities for improving the health of elderly people have been limited. This is due to a variety of factors: negative images of ageing and concepts that health promotion and disease prevention in old age are not worthwhile; lack of evidence of elderly people's ability to benefit from preventive and therapeutic interventions by their exclusion from epidemiological studies and clinical trials; and, until relatively recently, neglect by the research community of common problems of old age.

The goal of preventive strategies in old age includes not only improved survival but also the postponement or reduction of disability and a good quality of life.

The importance of healthy eating among elderly people

Old age is a period of increased vulnerability to poor nutrition. Eating behaviour may alter as a result of reduced income, social isolation, depression and dementia, while diseases and drugs may interfere with absorption.

Several studies have suggested that significant proportions of elderly people have undesirable nutritional intakes (Lehmann, 1989) even in communities with high levels of supplement use and moderate affluence. In elderly participants in the US Framingham Study 20% had folate and vitamin B_6 levels below recommended intakes (Sehlub et al., 1993). The Euronut Seneca study of 2500 75- to 80-year-old subjects in 19 European towns (the UK did not participate) found substantial proportions in some towns with low vitamin intakes, in particular, vitamin A and a high prevalence of serum B6 deficiency (Euronut SENECA investigators, 1991). Adverse over-nutrition was also a problem identified by this study; in nine towns the proportion with a body mass index over 30 kg/m^2 was 40 to 50%, and high mean cholesterol levels of up to 7 mmol/L were also found.

There are few data on the current nutritional status of elderly people in the UK. Surveys conducted in the 1960s and 70s found levels of gross malnutrition ranging from 3% to 7%, and very high levels reported for deficiencies of certain nutrients, especially riboflavin (24%), and vitamin C (31%). Vitamin D deficiency was reported in 7% (45).

A new cross-sectional dietary survey in people over 65 years in the UK has been undertaken (National Diet and Nutrition Survey) and will provide important updated information on dietary intakes and nutrient levels in elderly people (Finch et al., 1997).

Elderly people are classified on the basis of age (conventionally 65 years and over) but there is considerable heterogeneity within this age group, both in terms of age and other demographic and socioeconomic characteristics, health status, health beliefs and behaviours.

Living circumstances and household composition influence food purchasing, but additional factors such as levels of social support may also be important for the dietary behaviour of elderly people living alone. Availability of a car is lower in the elderly population, especially elderly women, and may limit access to food sources.

Variation in levels of physical and mental health in elderly people are also relevant since these factors influence the ability to access food services, prepare and enjoy food, as well as the metabolic consequences of ageing and disease on nutritional status.

Some of the barriers to the implementation of healthy lifestyles in the elderly include negative attitudes to changing behaviour and beliefs that they are too old to benefit from any such changes. This topic is considered in the parallel review *Opportunities for and barriers to change in the dietary behaviour of elderly people* (Lilley and Hunt, 1998).

Methodology and scope of the review

The present systematic review was conducted according to the guidelines set out in *Undertaking systematic reviews of research on effectiveness* (NHS Centre for Reviews and Dissemination, 1996). Electronic databases and key journals were searched, reference lists of reviews and other relevant articles were checked and key individuals and organisations were contacted in an attempt to locate published and unpublished studies for inclusion in the review. Articles identified in this way were then coded for inclusion or exclusion from the review according to certain eligibility criteria. The process of literature searching and the results of the search are described more fully in Appendices A–F. A standardised data extraction form was completed for all studies included in the review (see Appendix E). This included details of the study design, sample size, measurement tool validity, statistical techniques, response and withdrawal rates, major outcomes, generalisability, feasibility, and, where possible, reviewer-calculated estimates of effect size for each outcome. Judgements concerning study quality and intervention effectiveness were based on these and other criteria, and are summarised in the tables presented in Chapters 2 and 3. The published studies included in our review are considered separately according to the setting and context, on the assumption that the setting would influence both the type of nutrition intervention, its delivery and effectiveness.

Studies employing an experimental or quasi-experimental design were included in this review. That is, randomised controlled trials (RCTs), controlled non-randomised studies and also uncontrolled studies with pre- and post-intervention data. We also included two studies with post-intervention data only. Interventions were included if healthy eating was targeted specifically, or if there was a clearly defined nutritional component contained within a general health promotion package (i.e. as long as there were separate data relating to nutritional outcomes).

As well as including studies targeted specifically at elderly people (aged over 65) we sought to include interventions where elderly individuals were a sub-category of a broader population, providing data for elderly participants were reported separately and could be extracted for assessment. Studies were included where outcome measures consisted of diet-related physiological responses, dietary behaviour or dietary knowledge, attitudes and beliefs. Studies were excluded where individuals were specifically selected for being at high risk of disease, such as hypertension, hypercholesterolemia, obesity or family history of disease. Evaluations designed to prevent hypertension through healthy eating were also excluded since these have recently been reviewed elsewhere (Ebrahim and Davey Smith, 1996), but interventions to prevent obesity were included. Studies reporting the effect of mineral and vitamin supplementation were also excluded unless the intervention was designed to encourage the consumption of supplements as a healthy eating promotion.

Definitions

We defined *interventions* to promote healthy eating in the elderly to include: (i) nutrition education targeted at the individual or the community; (ii) individual counselling; (iii) policies to facilitate healthy eating behaviour but *not* the provision of meals. We defined *healthy eating* on the basis of UK guidelines for elderly people of the Committee on Medical Aspects of Food Policy (COMA) (Department of Health, 1992b) which stress avoiding under-nutrition in elderly people as well as recommendations similar to those for middle-aged and younger people aimed at reducing risk factors for cardiovascular disease (CVD). The COMA recommendations included: maintaining adequate energy intakes; reduction in non-milk extrinsic sugars; adopting diets to moderate cholesterol levels (including increasing oily fish consumption); reduced salt intake; increased consumption of fresh fruit, vegetables and wholegrain cereals. Additionally COMA recommended monitoring calcium levels, and consideration of vitamin D supplementation.

The COMA report, however, emphasised that the lack of research in many areas of nutrition in the elderly placed considerable restraints on the ability to make recommendations.

2. Reviewed studies

Nutrition interventions in elderly people in the community meal setting

Provision of meals in the community includes meals delivered to people's own homes, or in lunch clubs or day centres. In the UK meals delivered to people's homes are provided both by the voluntary sector and also by statutory services or the private sector with estimates of around 4% of people over-65 years living in the community receiving them (Davies, 1991). Meals in lunch clubs and day centres are provided from the voluntary sector with estimates of 3% of the over-65s receiving meals in this way. In the US provision of meals in the community was congressionally mandated through the 1972 and 1981 amendments to the 1965 Older Americans Act of 1965 which provided funding for both congregate sites and home delivered meals (Title III-C). The amendments also included the provision of nutrition education (a minimum of two sessions per year to programme participants).

While evaluation of the effectiveness of community meals settings in improving nutrition in elderly people is outside the scope of this review, the effectiveness of nutrition education conducted in the setting of community meals programmes is relevant. The setting is likely to include individuals at greatest nutritional 'risk' and the particular context of a community meal setting may enhance the effectiveness of a nutrition education intervention.

Published studies
Despite the US congressional mandate of nearly twenty years ago, and a large number of nutrition education initiatives, there have been extraordinarily few attempts to evaluate these. An evaluation of studies conducted in the period prior to this review found that nutrition education activities did not influence eating habits outside the programme (Kirschner Associates and Opinion Research Corporation, 1983).

Table D.1 in Appendix D gives the summary description of the three studies.

Design
Only one study is a randomised controlled trial, one is an experimental

controlled study but the method of allocation of the congregate meal sites to intervention or control is not described and is probably not random; the third study is an uncontrolled experimental design.

Design considerations

Size. All studies were extremely small ranging from 24 participants (Hermann *et al.*, 1990) to 66 (Mitic, 1985). Forty-four entered the non-randomised controlled study (Mayeda and Anderson, 1993) but no information on the distribution by group was given. No studies included any consideration of sample size or power and none presented 95% confidence intervals as an estimate of the possible range of effects.

Outcomes. Only one study (Hermann *et al.*, 1990) included objective measures of outcome (blood lipids). Blood pressure and anthropometry were also measured in this study but are liable to observer error which may be biased towards the intervention especially in an uncontrolled study. All studies used 24- or 48-hour dietary recall which may be susceptible to responder bias although some attempts to validate the responses were made in the RCT. The length of follow-up ranged from six weeks post intervention in the RCT (Mitic, 1985) to two months post intervention in the study by Mayeda and Anderson (1993), while in the study by Hermann *et al.* (1990) outcome data were collected immediately post intervention.

Withdrawals. A 34% default rate was reported in the study by Mayeda and Anderson (1993). In the other studies no data on withdrawals were reported so it is assumed that all subjects completed the study.

Statistical analysis. Mayeda and Anderson (1993) did not present the main outcome data and report only the lack of significant results. Allocation by cluster is not taken account of in their analysis.

Study contamination. The control group in the study by Mayeda received baseline nutrition surveys and food records which may have increased awareness of the intervention; the control group also received the programme at the end of the study so presumably had 'expectations' about the intervention.

Participants and setting

All studies were conducted in the US. Mitic's study mainly included people aged 65 to 74 years while only a wide age range (66–90) from the other two studies is presented. No breakdown by gender is given for Mitic's study but in the other two studies the majority (around 70%) were female. No details on ethnicity are given in any of the three studies.

Intervention

Content. The RCT (Mitic, 1985) specifically targeted individuals identified as having nutritionally inadequate diets. The intervention was aimed at improving the intake of eight essential nutrients (vitamins, minerals and protein). In contrast the interventions in the other two studies were aimed at reducing cardiovascular risk factors (fat, cholesterol and salt) and additionally included fitness information and a walk (Hermann *et al.*, 1990) or weight reduction programme (Mayeda and Anderson, 1993).

Method and intensity. Mitic's study, in particular, used the nature of the communal meals setting to enhance the intervention through group participation. The intervention appeared quite intensive over a four-week period although details of the length of each session and staff resources were not given. Hermann *et al.* (1990), while conducting more traditional didactic education, also used the setting to implement a daily walking programme. Their intervention consisted of 12 one-hour weekly classes conducted by a nutrition education specialist. The study by Mayeda and Anderson (1993) used postal education methods primarily, but also provided feedback on the analysis of individual food diaries. The intervention consisted of a single one-off postal package. No information is given on the resources required to carry out this activity.

Theoretical model. Mayeda and Anderson (1993) used the Health Belief Model and Acceptance of Change while Mitic (1985) used the model of Activated Health Education which emphasises motivation and responsibility.

Effectiveness
Both the RCT (Mitic, 1985) and the uncontrolled study (Hermann *et al.*, 1990) showed post-intervention benefits in outcome measures. Although the uncontrolled study was the only one to include objective measures and found changes in serum lipids compatible with effects of a small magnitude, the lack of a control group makes it difficult to attribute these to the intervention. The RCT found substantial changes in the intervention group measured by the proportion consuming at least 67% RDAs for each of eight nutrients. It is unlikely that such large benefits could be attributed to response bias. Both studies looked at short-term outcomes. The study by Mayeda and Anderson (1993) found no effects of the intervention but the study is seriously weakened by the lack of presentation of results, the large number of withdrawals and possible contamination of the control group.

Summary
Out of three published studies evaluating the effectiveness of a nutrition education programme in the context of community meals setting, only one study (Mitic, 1985) provided controlled and unconfounded evidence of the short-term benefits of the programme. Although response bias cannot be entirely discounted in this study, the large

improvements in nutrition can be attributed in part to the programme. The success of the intervention is likely to be related to: (i) the focus on high-risk individuals with nutritionally inadequate diets; (ii) the use of a motivational group-led model; (iii) the emphasis on improving vitamin, protein and mineral intakes. The results are likely to be generalisable to similar settings with individuals at high risk of nutritional deficiencies but longer-term benefits and cost-effectiveness need to be demonstrated.

Nutrition interventions in elderly people in communal settings

Evaluation of nutrition interventions in communal settings (other than community meals settings) includes studies conducted among residents of elderly housing projects or participating in an elderly community programme or attending a community centre. Studies in these settings have therefore primarily investigated the use of group settings as the context for nutrition education.

Published studies
Table D.2 in Appendix D gives the summary description of the nine studies.

Design
Three studies used a randomised control trial design (Bedell and Shackleton, 1989; Kupka-Schutt and Mitchell, 1992; Haber and Lacy, 1993); three studies had a control group but allocation was not random (Dennison et al., 1991, 1992; Rose, 1992) or was ambiguous (Higgins, 1988, 1989); and two studies used an uncontrolled experimental design (Doshi et al., 1994; Goldberg et al., 1989). The study by Constans et al. (1994) allocated people to intervention or control on the basis of their calcium intakes and hence the control group does not provide a meaningful comparison.

Design considerations
Size. The sample sizes were generally small, ranging from 15 per group (Bedell and Shackleton, 1989) to around 30 to 40 per group (Kupka-Schutt and Mitchell, 1992; Higgins, 1988, 1989; Doshi et al., 1994; Haber and Lacy, 1993; Dennison et al., 1992). Kupka-Schutt over-sampled the control group to allow for an expected high attrition rate. In the study by Rose (1992) the intervention was targeted informally at all residents in two housing units but only around a third participated in collection of data. Goldberg et al. (1989) presented data from 244 participants who had watched a quiz show video and completed pre- and post-intervention questionnaires but the total number of participants was not given.

No studies included consideration of sample sizes or study power in their study design and none presented 95% confidence intervals although Haber and Lacy (1993) presented 90% confidence intervals.

Outcomes. Two studies (Higgins, 1988, 1989; Doshi *et al.*, 1994) collected objective measures of nutrient intake in addition to dietary questionnaires. Higgins (1988, 1989) attempted to control for possible observer bias by masking control and intervention sites (though to what extent this was successful is doubtful). Several studies, used either 24-hour or three-day recall as a principal outcome measure along with questionnaires on nutrition knowledge or behaviour (Doshi *et al.*, 1994; Bedell and Shackleton, 1989; Kupka-Schutt and Mitchell, 1992) while other studies used only questionnaires on dietary knowledge or eating behaviours (Rose, 1992; Haber and Lacy, 1993; Goldberg *et al.*, 1989). The study by Constans *et al.* (1994) which focused on calcium intakes used seven-day food records only. For all self-reported measures, the possibility of respondent or observer bias cannot be discounted. Outcome data were collected either immediately or one week post intervention (Bedell and Shackleton, 1989; Dennison *et al.*, 1991, 1992; Haber and Lacy, 1993; Doshi *et al.*, 1994; Goldberg *et al.*, 1989) or six or eight weeks post intervention (Higgins, 1988, 1989; Kupka-Schutt and Mitchell, 1992). Rose (1992) collected outcome data three months after peer educators had been trained and Goldberg *et al.* (1989) four months after the video show. The longest period between intervention and outcome was two years, in the study by Constans *et al.* (1994). The validity of outcome measures was not discussed by most authors.

Withdrawals. In the study by Dennison *et al.* (1991, 1992), the initial intervention groups had 40 participants but nutrition outcome data were not available for 75% of these and for only 10 people in the control group, raising concerns about the original allocation and possible losses to follow up. Similarly in the study by Constans *et al.* (1994) 56% of participants did not participate in outcome collection and results were presented only for those with baseline and post-intervention data. Thirty-six per cent attrition occurred in the control group B only in the study by Kupka-Schutt and Mitchell (1992). Withdrawals were similar in both intervention and control in the study by Haber and Lacy (1993), around 11%.

Statistical analysis. Three studies (Dennison *et al.*, 1991, 1992; Higgins, 1988, 1989; Rose, 1992) allocated subjects to intervention or control according to housing site but did not take account of cluster allocation in the analysis. Three studies failed to test for between-group differences (Higgins, 1988, 1989; Kupka-Schutt and Mitchell, 1992; Constans *et al.*, 1994) although within-group changes were presented. Some studies presented only significant results from the food diaries (Dennison *et al.*, 1991, 1992) or results for the summary scores (Kupka-Schutt and Mitchell, 1992).

Study contamination. In all the RCTs the controls were either attending (Bedell and Shackleton, 1989) or were members of (Kupka-Schutt and Mitchell, 1992; Haber and Lacy, 1993), the same community programme as the intervention group.

Participants and setting

Eight studies were conducted in the US and one in France. The majority of participants in the US studies were female and white except the study by Doshi *et al.* (1994) which recruited only African Americans and that by Rose (1992) in which 70% were black. The average age was 75–76 years in three studies (Dennison *et al.*, 1991, 1992; Higgins, 1988, 1989; Rose, 1992), 72 years (Doshi *et al.*, 1994), predominantly aged 65 to 74 or mean age 68 years (Kupka-Schutt and Mitchell, 1992; Haber and Lacy, 1993; Constans *et al.*, 1994) while only the age ranges were given by Bedell and Shackleton (60–88 years) and Goldberg *et al.* (55–89).

Intervention

Content. In four studies the intervention was nutrition only while the studies by Higgins (1988, 1989), Rose (1992), and Haber and Lacy (1993) also included medical self-care, fitness and relaxation and Doshi *et al.* (1994) included fitness activities. In the study by Rose (1992) peer educators received training in CHD risk factors. In the study by Constans *et al.* (1994) the intervention was information to increase milk and dairy products in subjects with low calcium levels. Three studies included traditional instruction in nutrition (four basic foods and water) and two studies also included evaluation of individual food intake and setting of individual dietary goals (Kupka-Schutt and Mitchell, 1992; Dennison *et al.*, 1991, 1992) although the guidelines for these were not discussed. Doshi *et al.* (1994) focused on strategies to reduce high fat and sodium content of foods and Rose (1992) to reduce fat intake. The nutrition content of the intervention was not described in the study by Haber and Lacy (1993). The quiz show in the study by Goldberg *et al.* (1989) focused on weight control, food safety, dietary sodium and nutritional supplements.

Method and intensity. Bedell and Shackleton (1989) used didactic classes and handouts only. The other studies also used a variety of other methods: computer-assisted learning, cookery demonstrations (Doshi *et al.*, 1994), facilitator-led groups compared with lectures on dietary guidelines (Kupka-Schutt and Mitchell, 1992), peer educators (Rose, 1992), facilitator-led support groups and physician 'wellness prescriptions' (Haber and Lacy, 1993) while Higgins (1988, 1989) included social activities and group discussions. The study by Goldberg *et al.* (1989) used an innovative approach – that of a mock television quiz show. This was shown on video at local meetings of a retired persons' association. The 30-minute show used the format of a family competition compèred by a well-known comedian. The duration and frequency of the intervention was similar in several studies ranging from four one-hour sessions (Bedell and Shackleton, 1989; Dennison *et al.*, 1992; Kupka-Schutt and Mitchell, 1992), four two-and-a-half-hour sessions and four two-hour physical activities (Higgins, 1988, 1989), twice weekly sessions of unknown duration followed by 30 minutes' physical exercises (Doshi *et al.*, 1994). Peer educators were trained in eight two-hour sessions in the study by Rose (1992). Haber and Lacy (1993) used ten weekly didactic sessions of unknown duration followed by 30-minute group sessions with around 5 minutes per participant for completion of the wellness prescription by the physician.

Theoretical model. Kupka-Schutt and Mitchell (1992) followed Mitic's Nutrition Instruction model which emphasises motivation. Haber and Lacy (1993) emphasised the idea of behavioural contracts. Bedell and Shackleton (1989) used educational theory focusing on identifying educational needs and goal setting. Higgins (1988, 1989) emphasised learning through self-responsibility, decision-making and social support. Dennison *et al.* (1991, 1992) used a hands-on activated learning approach and the study by Rose (1992) was based on Social Learning Theory.

Effectiveness

The RCT by Bedell and Shackleton (1989) found large differences in nutrition knowledge in favour of intervention (compatible with moderate effect sizes) but these were not statistically significant and reflect the low power of the study ($n = 29$). Changes in dietary behaviour were minimal. The RCT by Kupka-Schutt and Mitchell (1992) showed significant benefits from both intervention and control A (received a simple didactic education programme) compared with control B (no education) in fat reduction but control group B had a high withdrawal rate and bias cannot be excluded. Intervention also improved the proportion with below recommended RDAs but this may have also led to some unfavourable trend in cholesterol and vitamin C levels. The RCT by Haber and Lacy (1993) found significant and large benefits (2- to 4-fold compared with control) in self-reported increases in fibre and reduction in sodium. Of the non-randomised controlled studies, the study by Dennison *et al.* (1991, 1992) found significant and large effects for both interventions (nutrition education with or without a computer) compared with control in fat intake but as these data only represent 25% of subjects originally allocated to intervention these results must be taken with extreme caution. A similar methodological weakness occurred in the study of peer educators by Rose (1992) which found a significant reduction in self-reported fat intake favouring the intervention sites but only a third of residents in the group participated in the study. The study by Higgins (1988, 1989) showed significant benefits of intervention on health and eating behaviours which were also reflected in reductions in cholesterol and increases in HDL cholesterol (although between group differences were not established). Similarly the uncontrolled study by Doshi et al. (1994) found significant reductions in total and LDL cholesterol compatible with effects of a small but important magnitude while waist circumference was also reduced. Calcium intakes improved in the intervention group in study by Constans et al. (1994). However as this group was selected for intervention on the basis of their low calcium intake and in the absence of an appropriate control group, the extent to which this can be attributed to the intervention remains uncertain. The video quiz show (Goldberg et al., 1989) produced more correct answers (up 25%) in a knowledge test (mainly concerning questions on weight control) but this had been reduced by around a half at the four-month re-test.

Summary

None of the nine studies conducted in the setting of community programmes or housing projects for the elderly provides adequate evidence for a benefit of intervention although conversely none of them provides adequate evidence for no benefit. The study by Dennison et al. (1991, 1992) suffered from serious methodological limitations while the RCTs by Bedell and Shackleton (1989) and Haber and Lacy (1993) were underpowered to detect even moderate effects on nutrition knowledge. The study by Doshi et al. (1994) found significant decreases in total and LDL cholesterol but in the absence of a control group these cannot be attributed to the intervention. The two RCTs that did demonstrate a benefit of intervention used the weaker outcomes of self-reported dietary behaviours. The non-randomised controlled study of Higgins (1988, 1989) showed quite impressive and favourable changes in cholesterol and HDL cholesterol compatible with the self-reported dietary changes but this study was not randomised and confounding and biased allocation may have occurred. The studies also differed in their results for the method of delivery of the intervention. In the RCT by Kupka-Schutt and Mitchell (1992), a nutrition education programme (with or without an intensive group-led approach) reduced self-reported fat intakes compared with a control group, while in Haber and Lacy's (1993) study the group receiving additional peer support and physician wellness prescriptions reported increased fibre intake and reduced sodium. The uncontrolled study by Goldberg et al. (1989) found improved knowledge in a rather narrow range of food-related questions following a video using the format of a television quiz show Although this was described as a mass media campaign the study could not address whether a television quiz show watched in the home environment would produce similar results to watching a video in a communal setting with the knowledge that an evaluation was taking place.

Taken together the studies provide weak evidence for improved eating behaviours in elderly people soon after nutrition or multifactorial interventions. Participants were mostly women but a range of income groups was represented across the studies. Most studies used the format of group-led activities which are less resource-intensive than individual counselling.

Nutrition interventions in the elderly population living in the community

This group of studies targeted elderly people in the community through a variety of methods. The studies used diverse strategies to deliver the interventions.

Published studies
Table D.3 in Appendix D gives the summary description of the six studies.

Design
None of the studies in this group used a randomised control design; two studies used a control group (Crockett et al., 1992; Egger et al., 1991). Of the four uncontrolled studies, one used a pre- and post-intervention design (Hackman and Wagner, 1990) and three were post-intervention surveys of a systematic sample of subjects targeted for the intervention (Weiss and Davis, 1985; Lach, Dwyer and Mann, 1994; Butler, Ohls and Posner, 1985).

Design considerations
Size. Study sizes ranged from around 300 for the two post-intervention surveys, around 100 in the uncontrolled experimental study (Hackman and Wagner, 1990). The study by Butler, Ohls and Posner (1985) surveyed 1684 people but no breakdown by the number of participants and non-participants was given. In both the controlled studies the method of allocation to type of intervention or control was at the community level but the method of allocation was not described. In the study by Crockett et al. (1992) there were 400 participants in total at baseline but the number by allocated group was not presented. The study by Egger et al. (1991) included three small towns of approximately 1500 population with a high proportion of retired residents.

No study discussed sample size or power in the consideration of study design.

Outcomes. None of the six studies included any objective measures of nutritional status – 24-hour recall was used by Butler, Ohls and Posner (1985). Food behaviour using food frequency questionnaires was measured in the studies which also collected pre-intervention data (Crockett et al., 1992; Hackman and Wagner, 1990) while the two post-intervention surveys focused on behavioural changes as a result of the intervention (a method likely to increase respondent bias). The community studies by Egger *et al.* (1991) used wholemeal and wholegrain bread sales (and laxative sales) over a two-week period both before and after the intervention.

Withdrawals. Sixteen per cent of subjects in the study by Crockett *et al.* (1992) did not return outcome data while in the study by Hackman and Wagner (1990) although no withdrawals were reported the amount of missing data ranged from zero for one community to around one-third in another community.

Statistical analysis. Descriptive data only were presented in two of the studies that collected only post-intervention data (Lach, Dwyer and Mann, 1994; Weiss and Davis, 1985) and did not include estimates of precision. The study by Crockett *et al.* (1992) did not take account of cluster allocation in the analysis and did not present any results for the major outcomes but only stated that there were no significant results.

Participants and setting

Five of the six studies were conducted in the US and one in Australia. The study by Crockett *et al.* (1992) only included subjects aged 60–70 with drivers' licences but the sample was probably representative of this group with around 60% females included. Egger's study was not exclusively in elderly people but in retirement communities. Other studies had similar age groups (mainly people in their late 60s or early 70s) and tended to over-represent women. Three studies were set in rural communities (Crockett *et al.*, 1992; Weiss and Davis, 1985; Egger *et al.*, 1991) and two in urban environments (Hackman and Wagner, 1990; Lach, Dwyer and Mann, 1994). The study by Butler *et al.* (1985) was conducted in low-income elderly.

Intervention

Content. Five studies were based on nutrition education. All of these studies included information to promote increased dietary fibre. The study by Egger *et al.* (1991) in the retirement communities in Australia concentrated exclusively on promoting consumption of wholemeal/wholegrain bread. Low fat diets were promoted in three studies (Crockett *et al.*, 1992; Weiss and Davis, 1985; Lach, Dwyer and Mann, 1994), low sodium in two (Weiss and Davis, 1985; Lach, Dwyer and Mann, 1994), increased calcium and dairy food intakes in two (Lach, Dwyer and Mann, 1994; Hackman and Wagner, 1990) and increased vitamins (Hackman and Wagner, 1990). Studies were often vague about the nutrition content of their intervention. The study by Butler, Ohls and Posner (1985) evaluated the Food Stamp programme which provided low-income elderly with either money or coupons to be exchanged for foods.

Method and intensity. Two studies used a print-based method to deliver the intervention, either through a free community seniors' newsletter (Weiss and Davis, 1985) or through a series of mailed information packs (Crockett *et al.*, 1992) with additional incentives and follow-up in the full intervention group (such as free cholesterol tests, shopping coupons). The community wholemeal bread promotion study (Egger *et al.*, 1991) compared a community organisation strategy (including the media, community events, bread pricing and social marketing) with a patient education system (leaflets handed out by local physicians). Hackman and Wagner's (1990) study was innovative in its use of garden boxes and instruction from master gardeners to encourage participants to grow their own vegetables. Nutrition classes using a lecture format with written handouts were also provided. In the study by Lach, Dwyer and Mann (1994) the intervention was delivered by written materials provided at stalls in supermarket, hospital and community settings and in partnership with food producers who also had exhibits. The intensity of the intervention varied considerably in the studies but often insufficient information was provided to fully assess the resources required. In particular the community organisation strategy in the wholemeal bread promotion study involved a range of participants and methods but these were not described (Egger *et al.*, 1991); similarly the supermarket study required support from volunteers, co-operation of supermarket and other staff but the level of resources required to deliver the intervention was not discussed. Even the study by Crockett *et al.* (1992) using an intervention of three mailed 'newsletters' also used follow-up phone calls, arrangements for free cholesterol tests, and food coupon incentives. The Gardening Project required the construction of garden boxes in individual households, bimonthly gardening and nutrition classes and home visits.

Theoretical model. Hackman and Wagner (1990) used a model of perception of control and social support.

Effectiveness

The study by Crockett *et al.* (1992) found no significant differences between the control and intervention groups in measures of food behaviour, dietary knowledge and purchasing habits. The data were only presented for some of the food frequency items and suggest that very small differences were observed (effect sizes of 0.2) which the study would not have power to detect. In the community study of wholemeal bread promotion, the community allocated to the community organisation strategy showed very large increases in wholemeal/wholegrain bread sales (of the order of a 50% increase) compared with either the community allocated to a patient education strategy or to the control community. Hackman and Wagner (1990) analysed the data separately by site in their uncontrolled study of gardening boxes. The data from the first site (the demonstration site) were more positive in showing changes in dietary habits based on food frequency questionnaires across a range of nutrients but the extension of the study to two low-income urban environments showed only increased water intake and dairy products with some possible adverse effects on some nutrients. Of the post-intervention studies, 17% reported changing their dietary behaviour (mainly increasing fibre intake and reducing sodium) in the study by Weiss and Davis (1985) of nutrition education in a seniors' newsletter while in the study of Lach, Dwyer and Mann (1994), following materials distributed in supermarket settings, 58% reported changes in dietary behaviour. Very small effects of the Food Stamp programme were found of which only calcium was significantly increased (Butler, Ohls and Posner, 1985).

Summary

Evidence for the effect of nutrition interventions targeting elderly people in the general community is poor. There are no RCTs in this group of studies and only two controlled studies. One of these controlled studies was somewhat different in that retirement communities rather than elderly individuals were targeted. No studies included objective measures of dietary behaviour although measurement of wholemeal/wholegrain bread sales is a close proxy to behaviour. The study by Crockett *et al.* (1992), although limited by non-random allocation, did use a systematic sample of elderly people with a high response rate and relatively low withdrawal rate. The study was of medium size for these types of studies (around 100 per group and more in the full intervention group). This study found no benefits from a low intensity mailed intervention in a rural community.

The most promising results were from the wholemeal bread study using a community strategy and focusing on only one food type. This study took place in a small community and may not be feasible in larger population settings. Although not discussed by the authors, it is likely that the intervention was resource intensive. Hackman and Wagner's (1990) study was uncontrolled and although some benefits from the programme may have occurred in changes in diet, these were not sustained across all sites. However the use of gardening boxes is an attractive one and deserves more rigorous evaluation. The post-intervention studies were weak methodologically, especially that of Lach, Dwyer and Mann (1994), with a response rate of 35%. It seems particularly surprising that these studies used such weak designs when a large effort was put into the interventions.

Nutrition interventions as part of health promotion interventions

Over the last twenty years there has been an increasing interest in disease prevention and health promotion among elderly people. Debate over whether improvements in life expectancy in elderly resulted in extra years of dependency and inactivity led to initiatives to promote health and reduce disability among older people. Health promotion strategies mostly included fitness and nutrition. While health promotion is clearly an important strategy for public health, the marketing of health promotion programmes also offers the potential for considerable financial gains. For example in the US health promotion programmes are sold as part of insurance schemes.

A number of demonstration studies of health promotion have been undertaken in the US but these earlier studies have rarely been evaluated. A fuller discussion of some of the better known of these studies is given in Chapter 5.

A US congressional mandate in 1986 (Consolidated Omnibus Reconciliation Act – COBRA) funded five studies to examine the cost-effectiveness of adding selected preventive services to Medicare benefits. These studies included the San Diego Medicare Preventive Health Project (Mayer et al., 1994; Elder et al., 1995) and the Rural Health Promotion Project (Ives, Kuller and Traven, 1993; Lave et al., 1996) which are reviewed below.

The three other studies funded under the scheme were excluded from the present review because there was neither a description of the nutrition component (other than as an area of individual counselling) nor nutrition outcomes. These studies include the North Carolina Medicare Program (Morrisey et al., 1995) and the Senior Health Watch carried out by John Hopkins (German et al., 1995) and the UCLA Medicare Screening and Health Promotion Trial (MSHPT) (Schweitzer et al., 1994). In all the COBRA studies the nutrition component was a small part of a very large battery of clinical procedures and examinations as well as preventive interventions including advice on smoking, alcohol, exercise, stress management, medication awareness and falls and accident prevention.

Published studies
The other group of studies included in the review, which were not funded under the COBRA recommendation, similarly included evaluation of a health promotion programme as part of insurance reimbursement. This group of studies (Leigh et al., 1992; Fries et al., 1992; Fries et al., 1993; Fries et al., 1994) evaluated one health promotion programme (the Senior Health Trac Program) offered to elderly people covered by the Blue Shield insurance company. The senior author and many of the co-authors of these studies had a financial interest either in Health Trac or in Blue Shield and these studies received financial support from Blue Shield. We also excluded a well-conducted randomised trial of a health promotion programme in British Columbia

(Hall *et al.,* 1992) as it was targeted at elderly people who had been assessed as in need of 'personal care at home'. Also the nutrition intervention was not described and was part of a large package including health promotion and social and physical assessment.

Table D.4 in Appendix D gives the summary description of the five studies.

Design

Four of the five studies were randomised controlled trials – the San Diego Medicare Preventive Health Project (Mayer *et al.,* 1994; Elder *et al.,* 1995), the Rural Health Promotion Project (Ives, Kuller and Traven, 1993; Lave *et al.,* 1996), the Bank of America Study (Leigh *et al.,* 1992; Fries *et al.,* 1993), with a similar trial in Blue Shield beneficiaries (Fries *et al.,* 1994). The fifth study was a prospective cohort study of Blue Shield beneficiaries receiving the Health Trac Program with concurrent baseline data from enrollees used as historical controls (Fries *et al.,* 1992).

Design considerations

Sample size. The trials were large, randomizing around 1,000 in each group in the San Diego study, the Rural Health Promotion Project and the Bank of America study. The trial in Blue Shield beneficiaries randomised around 34,000 of those in the Senior Health Trac Program to intervention and 1600 to control on the basis that it was desired to provide the programme to as many participants as possible (Fries *et al.,* 1994). The cohort study of Blue Shield beneficiaries receiving the Health Trac Program included 265,000 people (around 130,000 eligible for the Senior Health Trac Program) but around 30% were recent enrollees without follow-up data (Fries *et al.,* 1992). Thirty per cent of the elderly group were in the programme at the 12-month follow-up. Sample size calculations were not presented for the RCTs but it is likely that the studies did have adequate power to detect important differences. The cohort study was stated to have high power to detect differences of 1% at 0.01% alpha. In two studies eligibility or choice of the nutrition component meant that the actual numbers receiving the nutrition intervention was much smaller (around half in the Rural Health Promotion Project) and around a quarter in the San Diego study. This reduction in numbers would have consequences for study power.

Outcomes. The only study to include an objective measure of dietary behaviour was the Rural Health Promotion Project which measured blood cholesterol. The San Diego Project included body mass index but without details on how this was obtained (self-report or actually measured). Self-reported cholesterol data were available in the Bank of America and Blue Shield studies in around a quarter of participants. No attempts were made to validate these data. Both the San Diego and the

Bank of America and Blue Shield studies based their results for nutrition outcomes (and other risk behaviours) on self-report of types of food but with little discussion on the validity of their instrument. The Bank of America study presented test re-test data on the full health risk score and other measures of validity derived from responses in the lifestyle questionnaire but not on individual items apart from smoking.

Withdrawals. In the San Diego study 16% in the intervention group and 12% in the control group withdrew in the first year and just over 50% in both groups by the two-year follow-up. Blood cholesterol samples were not available in around a quarter of the intervention and control group in the Rural Health Promotion Project. In the Bank of America study 16% in both the intervention and control group had withdrawn by the first year and a further 15% by the end of the second year.

Statistical analysis. Apart from the Rural Health Promotion Project, most studies carried out a large number of statistical tests (especially in the Bank of America and Blue Shield studies) but without any consideration for multiple significance testing. Of particular concern is the use of one-sided statistical tests for the economic data in the Bank of America study (justified by the authors as a prior hypothesis). Because such a large battery of variables was used in these health promotion studies, questions on why some data items and not others were presented must also be raised. In the Bank of America study randomisation was by cluster but this was not taken into account in the analysis.

Participants and setting

All studies were conducted in the US: two in Medicare beneficiaries; one in retired employees of the Bank of America; and two in beneficiaries of Blue Shield insurance. The studies were thus predominantly in white low- to medium-income groups. The average age of participants was in the early 70s in the COBRA trials, and mid- to late 60s in the Bank of America and Blue Shield trials. The gender distribution in all trials slightly under-represented women, with women representing around 52% to 57% of trial participants.

Intervention

Content. All studies used a multifactorial risk assessment approach. In the Rural Health Promotion Project this included an initial screen to identify those with cholesterol above 240 mg/dl or overweight hypertensives for further counselling. However, only 40% to 50% of those eligible for counselling participated. The San Diego study used health risk assessment followed by individual counselling. Participants were only allowed to choose one goal from a hierarchy of health promotion activities which ranked physical activity first and nutrition second. Around a quarter chose a nutritional goal compared with 42% choosing a physical activity goal. Nutrition goals also allowed only one choice and were highly specific, for example increased cruciferous vegetable intake (chosen by 12%), reduced dietary fat (chosen by 8%), while only 2% chose decreased sodium or increased fibre. The Senior Health Trac Program used in the Bank of America and Blue Shield studies consisted of lifestyle questionnaires including dietary variables and other health behaviours such as smoking and alcohol intake.

Method and intensity. In the Rural Health Promotion Project participants were randomised to different reimbursement strategies – either fee for service or capitation – which meant that nutrition counselling was either delivered by hospital-based or home physician-based. No systematic protocol was provided but prior to the trial hospital nutritionists and dietitians and staff from physicians' offices were invited to training sessions on cholesterol lowering in the elderly. The San Diego study used trained student counsellors for individual goal setting with two telephone follow-ups in the first year. The Senior Health Trac Program was delivered entirely by post. Computerised feedback on individual questionnaires and recommendations were provided on the basis of returned lifestyle questionnaires at six-monthly intervals but no details are given on the resources required for this.

Theoretical model. Only the San Diego study specified a model of behaviour change – Kanfer's model of self-control and self-change, although the Bank of America studies emphasise the importance of self-sufficiency.

Effectiveness

The Rural Health Promotion Project, the only trial to use an objective measure of outcome, found no effect of nutrition counselling in reducing cholesterol levels. Although only a half of those eligible attended for nutrition counselling, cholesterol reduction did not differ between participants and non-participants. The results for weight reduction counselling were not reported. After one year in the trial, in the San Diego study a small effect of intervention on fat intake and also a small benefit for control on fibre intake was found but this had disappeared at the two-year follow-up. The Bank of America study showed favourable effects of intervention on a range of dietary habits when compared with the control group at 12 months. The Blue Shield studies also found favourable within-group changes but control data were not available.

Summary

The studies of nutrition interventions in the context of health promotion were generally well designed and of adequate size to detect important differences in nutrition outcomes (though with some exceptions as noted above). However, although the concept of including nutrition as part of a general package of health promotion is attractive there are a variety of problems which limit the findings from these studies: (i) a range of preventive strategies was included in a single package and it is, therefore, difficult to attribute benefits (if any) to any particular component of the package; (ii) the nutrition content of the intervention was poorly described; (iii) inadequate process data were presented for the nutrition component. As discussed above, several important trials of health promotion in elderly people had to be excluded from the review as there was no description of the nutrition intervention or nutrition outcomes.

With these caveats in mind, of the three RCTs with data available from a control group, only the Bank of America study found benefits across a wide range of healthy eating habits promoted by the intervention. The study used a six-monthly computerised feedback to a lifestyle questionnaire. The San Diego study used face-to-face counselling and goal setting but the restriction to only one goal limited the opportunity for a dietary benefit although a small reduction in dietary fat was found. It is worth noting that physical activity, the most popular choice for goal setting was significantly improved in the intervention group and this was maintained at the two-year follow-up. This result at least suggests that the intervention could change behaviour. The Rural Health Promotion Project adopted a pragmatic approach to cholesterol counselling which was not successful in changing cholesterol levels.

In summary, the evidence suggests that a feedback/goal-setting type intervention may lead to improved eating behaviours in elderly people but validation of self-reported changes is essential before uncritically accepting the benefits of such an approach.

3. Overview of reviewed studies

Design

Of the 23 studies, eight used a randomised control design, eight were controlled experimental studies, and seven were uncontrolled studies. The studies fall mainly into two groups: small studies with primarily nutrition-only interventions often undertaken in the setting of an elderly community programme (18 studies reviewed in Chapter 2, pp. 11–22) and large studies of multifactorial interventions in the context of adding health promotion to insurance policies (five studies reviewed in Chapter 2, pp. 22–27). We reviewed the studies in three different types of settings under the assumption that the setting would influence both the type of study and the intervention.

The first group of studies are the weakest methodologically but the nutrition interventions are usually well described. In contrast the second group of studies were mostly large randomised trials but the nutrition intervention was more likely to suffer from 'black box' effects reflecting the multifactorial nature of the intervention.

Outcomes

The majority of studies relied on self-reported diet behaviour. This ranged from 24-hour diet recall (six studies), food diaries, usually 2–3 day (four studies), food frequency questionnaires (two studies) and various other questionnaires on eating habits (eight studies). Only four studies measured blood cholesterol and of these only one was an RCT. Outcome data were collected very soon after the intervention apart from the health promotion studies (which included outcomes at least one year post intervention). Two studies had nutrition knowledge outcomes only.

Participants and setting

Of the 23 studies, 21 were carried out in the US, one in Australia and one in France. There were no studies from the UK. The age range of elderly people within the studies was very wide (often including people in their late 80s) but the implications of this both for appropriate nutrition guidelines and type of intervention were ignored. The health promotion studies tended to recruit middle income participants and the Bank of America/Blue Shield RCTs were exclusively in the retired workforce. The small community programme type studies were more likely to be skewed to low-income groups, and women.

Intervention strategy

The nutrition interventions used in the studies included:
(i) strategies to correct nutritional deficiencies in elderly people, for example to increase the proportion reaching RDAs, potential calcium deficiencies through increasing dairy food intakes;
(ii) strategies to reduce CVD risk factors, for example lower fat intakes, less sodium, calorie control, increased fibre;
(iii) poorly defined strategies, i.e. the content of the intervention was described but its purpose was not, for example basic four foods and water, nutritional needs of ageing.

Clearly the first strategy could have adverse effects on the second and conversely if these were not properly targeted. Studies that used individual food records with feedback and personal goal-setting would be most likely to avoid this. However studies did not report outcomes in sufficient detail to be able to assess this.

Table 3.1 shows the results for the studies grouped according to the nutrition strategy. The Food Stamp programme is a policy evaluation and is not included in the table. This programme, which specifically targeted low-income elderly, found no impact of the intervention, but this was a cross-sectional study and therefore not an adequate evaluation. The studies stressing basic nutritional needs have tended to be small studies and all of them were appropriately conducted within settings where participants might be at high risk of nutritional deficiencies. Of the two RCTs one showed significant improvements, the other had no effect. Both studies were small but the study with the positive effect targeted those with intakes below RDAs. Although the study by Higgins (1988, 1989) appeared to focus on basic nutritional needs, favourable changes in body weight and cholesterol were found but as the study used non-random allocation to control, the evidence for the apparent benefits is weakened.

Two studies concentrated on one specific nutrient or food. Both studies showed favourable intervention effects in comparison with a control group. Neither study used random allocation and the study on calcium intake used an inappropriate control group.

The most popular nutrition strategy was CVD risk factor modification focusing on fat and salt intake, weight control and increased fibre. Of the three large RCTs in this group, decreased fat intake (based on lifestyle questionnaires) was found in two studies but the only study to measure blood cholesterol found no differences between intervention and control. One small well-conducted RCT in this group found increased fibre and decreased sodium based on food questionnaires. Most of the other studies that used a CVD modification strategy were of poor quality either due to design faults, or high withdrawals.

In a few studies the nutrition strategy was unclear. All these studies had methodological problems or inadequate outcomes.

Delivery of intervention

These ranged from traditional class-based didactic sessions to individual feedback and goal-setting either through postal questionnaires or through peer group or individual counselling sessions. Table 3.2 shows the studies by method of delivery.

Small group education methods were associated with a successful intervention in two out of three reasonable quality but small studies. Although the study by Higgins (1988, 1989) used traditional group teaching, social and physical activities were also included and may have improved group cohesion and motivation. None of these studies reported withdrawals. Education using the printed media was the method of delivery of the intervention in four studies, two of which used a controlled design. In the study by Mayeda and Anderson (1993) there was a high withdrawal rate and no effects of the intervention while the study by Crockett et al. (1992) had a high return of outcome data but no effects due to the intervention. Of the well-conducted studies, individual diet feedback and goal-setting was used in seven studies, six of them RCTs (one with no control dietary outcomes). Two of these RCTs also used group-based education classes. One-to-one counselling was used by three RCTs and associated with a positive intervention in two. The study which found no benefit, the Rural Health Promotion Project used a loose counselling intervention. Small group feedback was used in one small RCT which found intervention benefits. The Bank of America and Blue Shield studies used postal questionnaires with computerised feedback which were associated with benefits in improved dietary habits.

Other studies used innovative methods. Dennison et al. (1991, 1992) used computer-assisted education including analysis of personal food diaries, but possible lack of enthusiasm for this method is suggested by the large amount of missing outcome data. Similarly Rose (1992) trained peer educators in elderly housing units with informal dissemination to residents but less than a third of residents participated in data collection, suggesting lack of impact of educators although self-reported fat intake did decrease compared with a non-random control group. Goldberg used a television quiz show video and found improved knowledge after the show but there were no behavioural measures. The community organisation strategy to promote wholemeal bread was superior to a patient leaflet and a control group and produced large effects. The gardening box scheme along with instruction in nutrition and gardening was not a controlled study but suggested that possible benefits were site-specific.

Summary

There is some limited evidence primarily from two large and two small RCTs that a nutrition intervention in elderly people can produce benefits in self-reported dietary behaviours. There is no evidence of a benefit on blood cholesterol and the only large well-conducted RCT which measured this outcome found no differences between intervention and control. A variety of reasons could have contributed to this lack of effect, primarily low uptake and a weak counselling strategy. In three of the four positive RCTs the interventions were CVD risk-based and used a strategy of individual feedback and goal-setting to produce reductions in fat intake (two studies), reduced salt (two studies), and increased fibre (two studies). The other positive RCT targeted low-income inner city elderly with poor nutrition intakes and used a group education approach to produce very large benefits in improved minimum nutrition requirements. The four positive studies were conducted in the US. Of the two small RCTs one was conducted in the setting of communal eating programmes and the other in attenders at a local geriatric community programme. It is likely that these results are generalisable to similar settings in the UK. The two large RCTs of health promotion linked to health insurance may not be generalisable to the UK. Moreover the costs and resources to deliver the health promotion package are likely to be very different in the UK.

Table 3.1. Studies grouped by type of intervention strategy

Intervention strategy	Authors	Study design	Intervention effect	Reviewers' comments
Basic nutritional needs	Mitic, 1985	Randomised controlled trial	Large effects on food diary RDAs.	Small, well conducted study.
	Higgins, 1988/ Higgins, 1989	Experimental controlled	10% decreased cholesterol, body weight; 20% increased HDL.	Well conducted small study. Bias due to non-random allocation.
	Bedell and Shackleton, 1989	Randomised controlled trial	No significant effects.	Small study underpowered to detect observed moderate effects.
	Hackman and Wagner, 1990	Uncontrolled experimental	Improved intakes in 1/3 sites only.	Innovative gardening study, but no control.
One specific food / nutrient	Egger et al., 1991	Experimental controlled	Increase in wholemeal/wholegrain bread sales.	Well conducted study. Possible bias due to non-random allocation.
	Constans et al., 1994	Experimental controlled	Increase in dietary calcium.	Inappropriate control group.
CVD risk factor modification	Weiss and Davis, 1985	Uncontrolled experimental	Limited effect on changing diets.	Cannot be assessed. No pre-intervention data.
	Crockett et al., 1992	Experimental controlled	No effects.	Well conducted study. Possible bias due to non-random allocation.
	Fries et al., 1992	Cohort	Favourable changes in fat and salt intake.	Some control for secular trends.
	Leigh et al., 1992/ Fries et al., 1993	Randomised controlled trial	Around 10% improved dietary habits: fat, salt, wholegrain bread, according to self-report data.	Well conducted study.
	Rose, 1992	Experimental controlled	Decreased self-reported fat intake.	Low participation in outcome collection.
	Haber and Lacy, 1993	Randomised controlled trial	Increased fibre and decreased sodium (food questionnaire).	Small well conducted study.
	Ives, Kuller and Traven, 1993/ Lave et al., 1996	Randomised controlled trial	No effects on blood cholesterol.	Well conducted study, but vague strategy.
	Mayeda and Anderson, 1993	Experimental controlled	No effects.	Small study. High withdrawal rate.
	Doshi et al., 1994	Uncontrolled experimental	Reduced total and LDL cholesterol.	Cannot be attributed to intervention.
	Fries et al., 1994	Randomised controlled trial	Favourable trends in fat intake in intervention group.	No control data for dietary outcomes.
	Lach, Dwyer and Mann, 1994	Uncontrolled experimental	58% reported dietary change.	Poor response rate and no pre-intervention data.

Table 3.1. Studies grouped by type of intervention strategy (contd)

Intervention strategy	Authors	Study design	Intervention effect	Reviewers' comments
Both basic nutritional need and CVD risk factor modification	Hermann et al., 1990	Uncontrolled experimental	Favourable effects on blood lipids.	Cannot be attributed to intervention.
	Mayer et al., 1994/ Elder et al., 1995	Randomised controlled trial	Small effects on fat intake. Increase in fibre intake in controls.	Well conducted study. Limitation of strategy of one health promotion goal only.
Uncertain	Goldberg et al., 1989	Uncontrolled experimental	Improved performance on knowledge questionnaire.	Limited relevance of food knowledge. No behavioural measures.
	Dennison et al., 1991/Dennison et al., 1992	Experimental controlled	Decreased saturated fat (food diary).	Very poor study. Missing outcomes in 75%.
	Kupka-Schutt and Mitchell, 1992	Randomised controlled trial	Small effect on food diary intake.	Possible bias due to high withdrawal in controls.

Table 3.2. Studies grouped by delivery of intervention

Intervention strategy	Authors	Study design	Intervention effect	Reviewers' comments
Education/information				
(i) Small group	Mitic, 1985	Randomised controlled trial	Large effects on food diary RDAs.	Small, well conducted study.
	Higgins, 1988/ Higgins, 1989	Experimental controlled	10% decreased cholesterol, body weight; 20% increased HDL.	Well conducted small study. Bias due to non-random allocation.
	Bedell and Shackleton, 1989	Randomised controlled trial	No significant effects.	Small study underpowered to detect observed moderate effects.
	Hermann et al., 1990	Uncontrolled experimental	Favourable effects on blood lipids.	Cannot be attributed to intervention.
(ii) Print media	Doshi et al., 1994	Uncontrolled experimental	Reduced total and LDL cholesterol.	Cannot be attributed to intervention.
	Weiss and Davis, 1985	Uncontrolled experimental	Limited effect on changing diets.	Cannot be assessed. No pre-intervention data.
	Crockett et al., 1992	Experimental controlled	No effects.	Well conducted study. Possible bias due to non-random allocation.
	Mayeda and Anderson, 1993	Experimental controlled	No effects.	Small study. High withdrawal rate.
	Lach, Dwyer and Mann, 1994	Uncontrolled experimental	58% reported dietary change.	Poor response rate and no pre-intervention data.
Individual diet feedback and goal setting				
(i) One-to-one	Ives, Kuller and Traven, 1993/ Lave et al., 1996	Randomised controlled trial	No effects on blood cholesterol.	Well conducted study, but vague strategy.
	Constans et al., 1994	Experimental controlled	Increase in dietary calcium.	Inappropriate control group.
(ii) Small group	Kupka-Schutt and Mitchell, 1992	Randomised controlled trial	Small effect on food diary intake.	Possible bias due to high withdrawal in controls.
(iii) Print media	Fries et al., 1992	Cohort	Favourable changes in fat and salt intake.	Some control for secular trends.
	Leigh et al., 1992/ Fries et al., 1993	Randomised controlled trial	Around 10% improved dietary habits: fat, salt, wholegrain bread, according to self-report data.	Well conducted study.
	Fries et al., 1994	Randomised controlled trial	Favourable trends in fat intake in intervention group.	No control data for dietary outcomes.

Table 3.2. Studies grouped by delivery of intervention (contd)

Intervention strategy	Authors	Study design	Intervention effect	Reviewers' comments
Both education and feedback (one-to-one)	Hader and Lacy, 1993	Randomised controlled trial	Increased fibre and decreased sodium (food questionnaire).	Small well conducted study.
	Mayer et al., 1994/ Elder et al., 1995	Randomised controlled trial	Small effects on fat intake. Increase in fibre intake in controls.	Well conducted study. Limitation of strategy of one health promotion goal only.
Others				
(i) Quiz show video	Goldberg et al., 1989	Uncontrolled experimental	Improved performance on knowledge questionnaire.	Limited relevance of food knowledge. No behavioural measures.
(ii) Gardening boxes and education diaries	Hackman and Wegner, 1990	Uncontrolled experimental	Improved intakes in 1/3 sites only.	Innovative gardening study, but no control.
(iii) Community organisation	Egger et al., 1991	Experimental controlled	Increase in wholemeal/wholegrain bread sales.	Well conducted study. Possible bias due to non-random allocation.
(iv) Computer assisted	Dennison et al., 1991/Dennison et al., 1992	Experimental controlled	Decreased saturated fat (food diary).	Very poor study. Missing outcomes in 75%.
(v) Peer educators	Rose, 1992	Experimental controlled	Decreased self-reported fat intake.	Low participation in outcome collection.

4. Nutrition interventions in the general population

Healthy eating interventions in the community which were not specifically targeted at elderly people have been reviewed elsewhere (Roe *et al.*, 1998). Of the 76 studies reviewed, 36 excluded participants over 65 years; a further 16 studies gave no upper age range, but given the average age of participants it is unlikely that these included any over 65 years; 21 addressed whole communities, consumers or work sites and may have reached a proportion of individuals over the age of 65, but no data were given; and 3 definitely included a number of participants over 65 years, but there was no breakdown of the results by age.

The influence of age on some outcomes, such as compliance with the study protocol have been reported by some studies and are briefly reviewed here.

The Pawtucket Heart Health program SCORE included a randomised trial of methods to enhance compliance with dietary recommendations in participants with elevated cholesterol levels. In an analysis of factors predicting compliance, older people were less likely to report making dietary changes (Gans *et al.*, 1994). The mean age in this study was 51 years with around 10% aged 65+. However an earlier small survey from the programme found similar proportions reporting change in diet or physician attendance although older people were more likely to have been told by their physician that their cholesterol values were not a problem; older people were less likely to recall their actual blood cholesterol value. The Massachussets Screening Project found that participation rates by elderly people aged 70 and over were around half that expected but slightly better than expected for those aged 60–69 years. In this study compliance with referral to a physician increased with increasing age. In the control cities of the Stanford Five City study those aged 50–74 years at baseline had similar or even greater falls in cholesterol over the decade from 1980 to 1990 as did younger adults (Frank *et al.*, 1992). In the intervention cities of the Stanford Five City Project older age (55 to 74 years) was the most important determinant of a positive change in a CVD risk factor score (Winkleby, Flora and Kraemer, 1994).

5. Studies not included or in progress

Continuing or well known studies without adequate evaluation

We excluded published studies where, although an evaluation of a nutrition intervention had been carried out, this was inadequately described. In addition we were unable to find a published evaluation of some well known health promotion and nutrition intervention projects in the elderly because they were reported only at the demonstration stage and did not proceed to a full evaluation. Some of these studies are described here.

The Dartmouth Self Care Program for Senior Citizens (Nelson *et al.*, 1984; Simmons *et al.*, 1989) is a community self-care programme which includes medical self-care education, nutrition, exercise and relaxation as well as knowledge of social services. The study has been tested using communities in New Hampshire and Miami in 147 elderly persons in the intervention group and 104 in the control group. Pre- and post-intervention outcomes were based on self-reported attempts to change lifestyle including nutrition and weight loss and measured immediately after the intervention (at 3 months) and then at one year. At 3 and 12 months significantly more elderly people in the intervention group reported changes in nutrition (55% and 48%) compared with control (22% and 27%) and weight loss (56% and 50%) in intervention and 32% and 37% in control at the 3- and 12-month points respectively. Similar results favouring intervention were found for self-reported changes in physical exercise and tension. More objective measures of health-care utilisation and health status did not differ between the groups. There were some subgroup analyses in favour of quality of life improvements in the intervention group. The authors concluded that the programme was successful and that medical care self-education can increase the capacity of the elderly to manage their health. The perceived success of the Dartmouth Program led to its successor, the Staying Healthy after Fifty (SHAF) Program which has been widely implemented through the US. No further evaluation has been found for this study.

The Growing Younger Program (Kemper, 1986) is a non-profit health promotion programme which includes nutrition and simple self-care medical education, cardiovascular risk factor reduction, and social interaction. It has clearly defined quantitative objectives. The programme has a strong social content including parties, walks and friendship circles. A large number of health professionals and volunteers are involved in the programme which is set in the town of Boise Idaho and has over 10% of adults over 60 years recruited to the programme. Evaluation is based on six-monthly changes from baseline in self-reported health behaviours, biometric data (including body weight, blood pressure and cholesterol). Only very preliminary results were published in 1986.

The Tenderloin Senior Outreach Program (TSOP) started in 1979 as a health behaviour programme set in a high crime, low socioeconomic San Francisco community which also has a high proportion of single elderly people mainly living in hotels (Wechsler and Minkler, 1986). TSOP is directed at these low-income elderly residents. Support groups are held in the hotels facilitated by students in public health to help improve basic nutrition, reduce alcohol consumption and increase exercise. In 1983 TSOP participants identified access to good food as their main barrier to healthy eating and a range of initiatives were set up (such as a local hotel minimarket selling fresh produce at cost), or being planned (such as community kitchens) at the time of publication. TSOP became a non-profit agency in 1982 with funding support. No further evaluation has been found for this study.

The Wallingford Wellness Project was a 3-year controlled community-based health promotion program for the elderly (Lalonde and Fallcreek, 1985). The intervention included physical fitness classes including aerobics, stress management and nutrition. The nutrition component focused on healthy low-cost eating to achieve a balanced diet low in fat, sugar, salt and cholesterol. The project was directed at the whole community although the main research interest was in middle-aged and elderly people. The experimental group consisted of 90 people aged 55 years and over with an average age of 70 years and a comparison group of 44 people with an average age of 73 years. Both the experimental and control groups were mainly women. A large number of measures were collected at baseline and 6 months after the end of the 21-week intervention. Within-group changes in 'behavioural change' related to nutrition only were reported for the nutrition outcomes and these were found to be significantly improved in the intervention group but not the control group. Results of the two-year follow-up using mailed questionnaires and a large number of variables have also been published but only as summary variables. Healthy eating lifestyle habits relating to nutrition were maintained in the experimental group but not for health information (Lalonde, Hooyman and Blumhagen, 1988). No further evaluation has been found for this study.

The Sun Cities Study, a controlled intervention testing a computerised feedback on health education derived from Health Watch, a large longitudinal study of aging was excluded as the results had only been published in abstract form (Schmidt, 1990).

Grey literature in the UK

Consultation with key organisations and individuals provided the reviewers with details of a number of relevant unpublished projects. These can be divided into UK projects, which are presently described, and a project from Australia which is described in the section following this.

Although there were no published British studies eligible for inclusion in the present review, grey literature contacts provided descriptions of several small-scale, completed or continuing health promotion projects targeting the elderly in the UK. Most of these are demonstration projects. They give some indication of the local initiatives being carried out across the UK to promote healthy eating, but are *not* designed to evaluate the interventions.

The Ageing Well Initiative is a national health promotion programme managed by Age Concern and supported by the Department of Health, the Health Education Authority, Merck Sharpe & Dohme Ltd and Private Patients Plan Ltd. Launched in 1993, the aim of this programme was to 'promote effective models of healthy ageing', using peer group health volunteers (Senior Health Mentors) and a wide variety of health promotion activities, including healthy eating. Nine pilot projects were set up across the UK, using Senior Health Mentors to give support and advice to older people about their health. A government-funded evaluation of this national programme has not yet been published and was not available for this review. The number of projects including nutrition advice and support is unknown. However, a local evaluation of one of the projects in Wales, 'The Barry Senior Health Shop' is described below (F. Hunt, personal communication).

The focus of the Barry Senior Health Shop project is a healthy eating snack bar (Senior Health Shop), designed to encourage individuals above the age of 50 to look after themselves through a healthy diet, suitable exercise, activities and relaxation. An evaluation of the Senior Health Shop activities consisted of a self-completed questionnaire distributed to shop customers in 1994 ($n = 48$) and 1995 ($n = 74$). Individuals visiting the shop were mostly aged between 60 and 80 years, with just over half being female. Although most customers came to the shop for a snack and tea or coffee, the numbers picking up health information rose from 14 (29%) to 29 (39%) from 1994 to 1995. Two-thirds of customers said that visiting the shop had made them think about taking action in relation to some aspect of their health, particularly healthy eating.

In addition to the nine pilot projects undertaken, a further generation of locally funded projects are under way in the UK. There is also a European network with continuing projects in France, Germany, Greece, Ireland, Italy, the Netherlands, Portugal and Spain.

Promoting Healthier Eating in Wood End, Coventry aimed to provide nutrition education for a small number of elderly people in a semi-sheltered, independent housing complex. This took the form of four two-hour practical sessions as requested by residents for cookery practicals and recipe ideas. At the end of each practical, residents reported their like or dislike for each recipe and whether or not they would cook it at home. Most answered in the affirmative for both questions. When asked to identify a change made as a result of attending the course, responses included incorporating greater variety and ideas into cookery and reducing fat levels in cooking.

Castlemilk Food Co-op Development Project, Glasgow. The aim of the Castlemilk project is to develop and maintain food cooperatives throughout Castlemilk, Glasgow. Although Healthy Castlemilk targets the entire age range in the community, there have been specific interventions directed towards elderly individuals.
Healthy eating promotions have included:

(a) Work with community cafés (the Pensioners Action Centre) to promote healthy food.
(b) Production of a recipe book with simple, cheap and nutritious recipes relevant to local needs.
(c) 'Winter Warmers' promotion for Castlemilk pensioners. In conjunction with Kwik Save, pensioners were given vouchers for £1 off their shopping bill for the purchase of certain non-perishable goods (hot drinks, hot meals and dessert), to encourage them to build up a 'store cupboard' for winter emergencies. Over 600 pensioners took part in this promotion.

Feedback obtained from the individuals benefiting from these health promotion activities has been positive. For example, a pensioner taking part in the Winter Warmers promotion commented 'I've never thought of having a winter store before and used to sit in the house and worry if the weather was bad or I wasn't feeling well, how I would manage to the shops, now I can relax knowing . . . I have food in the cupboard'.

Look After Yourself at the Terry Dowling Centre, Wythenshawe, Manchester. This health promotion campaign was run by the Manchester Health Promotion Service and supported by the Health

Education Authority and the Department of Health. The Look After Yourself (LAY) project was targeted at users of the Terry Dowling Centre in Wythenshawe, who were at least 60 years old. The course consisted of exercise promotion, a relaxation programme and a number of health objectives, including healthy eating. Courses were run by qualified tutors for a small number of elderly people, and comprised an average of ten weekly sessions of two hours' duration. Each health topic had specific objectives based on changes in knowledge, skills learnt, contribution to helping with a problem or meeting a need. These were evaluated during each session and at the end of the whole course using a questionnaire. Feedback from the course participants was positive for all aspects of the course. With respect to the nutrition component, respondents reported that they had learnt recipes for healthy dishes, had more ideas for cooking dishes for one person and had learnt to avoid binge eating.

The Barri Grubb Food Project is a healthy eating promotion targeted at the local population of Greater Pilton, Edinburgh. Funded by the Edinburgh Healthcare (NHS) Trust in an area of urban deprivation, the project tackles three main barriers to healthy eating: health food cost, availability and education. Healthy food is sold at cost price from the Barri Grubb shop (based at Pilton Community Health Project), through local deliveries and by sales from the Barri Grubb van. Fresh fruit, vegetables, pasta, cereals and oil-rich fish are therefore supplied to the local community in an accessible, affordable way. In addition, local taster sessions and cookery demonstrations are undertaken in an educational capacity to raise awareness of the relationship between healthy eating and health.

An independent evaluation of the project was carried out in 1994. Barri Grubb produce was found to be considerably cheaper than local retail produce, and all the customers interviewed reported an increased uptake of fruit and vegetables since using Barri Grubb. On the basis of self-completed questionnaires completed over a four-week period, 10% of the customers attending the Barri Grubb shop were found to be aged 65 years or older.

Nutrition screening initiatives – work in progress

In addition to the UK studies described above, the grey literature search uncovered an Australian project using the Australian Nutrition Screening Initiative (ANSI), which was launched in June 1994. This screening tool was designed to provide warning signs for nutritional risk among independent older people, and trigger the individual or carer to take steps to improve nutrition if necessary. The Central Coast Area

Health Service (CCAHS) decided to use ANSI as part of a community project to highlight nutrition issues targeting older people. In consultation with over 200 home carers and a range of health professionals, the CCAHS produced a booklet called *Reduce the risk: a commonsense guide to preventing poor nutrition in older people* (Bunney and Bartl, 1996). The booklet translates the issues highlighted by ANSI into practical ideas, advice and suggestions for improving nutritional status. The booklet was designed to be of value to both older people themselves, and service providers. It has received a positive response from the National ANSI Committee and other government bodies.

Similar continuing research based on the US Nutrition Screening Initiative (NSI) (Posner *et al.*, 1993) is under way in the United States. Many American studies currently use the NSI to identify elderly individuals at nutritional risk, although resulting health promotion interventions with evaluated outcomes are yet to be published. However, there is some concern that an emphasis on nutritional *deficiency* in the NSI checklist may lower detection of problems related to over-eating with resulting limitations for its use as a health promotion tool (Contento *et al.*, 1995).

6. Conclusions and recommendations

Conclusions

Our search revealed a large literature on nutrition interventions in the elderly and a paucity of evaluative studies. It seems that this is an area where there is much enthusiasm but very little evidence. We have described in Chapter 5 a number of studies of health promotion/nutrition interventions in the elderly which are being disseminated but have not been evaluated or where the evaluation is inadequate. New developments in nutrition interventions such as nutrition screening initiatives in the US and Australia described in Chapter 5 are currently being evaluated but no detailed results were published within the period covered by this review. We identified one other recent review of nutrition education in elderly people (Contento *et al.*, 1995). Although this review gave an interesting overview of methods and models of nutrition education, there was no critical appraisal of the studies reviewed.

We identified only 23 studies which met our criteria and which included some description of the nutrition intervention and nutrition outcomes. We accepted some study designs that would not be capable of providing good scientific evidence because we wanted to provide a comprehensive picture of the range and quality of such 'evaluative' studies that have been undertaken. Publication bias may well be a problem especially for small 'negative' studies. In the abstracts and conclusions of most of the studies reviewed, the authors were positive about the benefits of nutrition intervention even when the results of their studies were equivocal or negative or when the study design might have suggested more caution. Many small studies were conducted by single or dual authors suggesting limited resources had been committed to the studies. In contrast, the multifactorial health promotion studies which were conducted in the context of health insurance were large, long-term, high resource studies.

There were serious design faults in many of the studies reviewed. Most commonly they were small and underpowered; used a non-random control group or were uncontrolled; and relied on self-reported data, mostly with no attention to validity of outcome measures . A few studies had high withdrawal rates or missing data and many used inappropriate statistical analyses. None of the seven studies that used cluster allocation or randomisation employed the appropriate method of analysis.

Most studies used nutritional interventions to reduce CVD risk with an emphasis on low fat intakes, reduced salt and increased fruit and vegetables. Six studies used strategies to correct nutritional deficiencies in elderly people while two other studies appeared to combine both approaches. The strategy of the intervention was unclear in three others. This highlights an important difference between nutritional interventions in elderly people and those in middle age and younger populations. Elderly people are a heterogeneous group and include people with nutritional deficiencies, and those at risk of nutritional deficiencies, as well as those with adequate diets. Interventions promoting low fat, low calorie diets and weight reduction may therefore be undesirable in some elderly people. Assessing individual dietary intake before promoting the appropriate nutritional intervention is an area which requires more attention.

Moreover it cannot be assumed that recommendations and interventions for healthy eating for elderly people are similar to those at younger ages. Surveys of nutrition in the elderly have tended to use recommended daily intakes (RDIs) as the criterion. The proportion of elderly people falling outside RDIs is, however, of limited value since RDIs are uncertain for elderly people. Moreover RDIs reflect the nutritional requirements needed to maintain physiological function rather than the optimal intakes to maintain health and prevent disease. Dietary guidelines which more specifically address the prevention of disease and disability in populations, are derived from longitudinal studies which to date have been conducted primarily in middle-aged people. There is far less evidence to inform nutritional recommendations for elderly people, in particular very elderly people. The acceptance and endorsement of healthy eating guidelines for elderly people by public health practitioners requires a stronger body of scientific evidence.

Our review provided limited evidence for the effectiveness of healthy eating interventions in elderly people. Two large positive trials which included nutrition as part of general health promotion showed some benefits but the setting of the intervention in the context of the US health insurance scheme limits the applicability to the UK. These studies used interventions promoting healthy eating behaviours to reduce CVD risk (especially lower fat intake). Two small studies in the setting of community programmes for elderly people also showed benefits; one of these studies specifically targeted elderly people at high risk of nutritional deficiencies while the other study used a multifactorial CHD risk approach. None of these four studies had objective measures of outcome, and relied on self-reported dietary behaviour.

There was a wide age range of elderly people but most studies did not have the power to examine differential effects of interventions with age. The exception to this was the RCT of the Blue Shield Insurance group.

Changes in eating behaviours were similar in a younger elderly group (average age 63 years) to an older group (average age 73 years) but dietary results were not reported for the control group.

Although elderly people have been included in some of the large controlled studies of healthy eating interventions in the general community as discussed in Chapter 4, few studies have published separate analyses by age and it is likely that such a subgroup analysis would be low powered. Such studies that have investigated the effects of age have generally found that older age was not a barrier to dietary change.

We found only a handful of studies that examined either policy or strategies directed at the entire community. The results of the study by Butler, Ohls and Posner (1985) suggest that the Food Stamp Program did not lead to an improvement in diet. Other studies on the Food Stamp Program have been published either before the period covered by this review or as survey data only. These studies generally reach similar conclusions to those of Butler, Ohls and Posner. The non-randomised controlled study conducted in Australia evaluated a community organisation strategy which included bread pricing policy as well as social marketing and media communication (Egger *et al.*, 1991). The results suggested a very large benefit from this strategy with a 50% increase in wholemeal/wholegrain bread supplies but the level of resources and effort required may be considerable.

Most studies have been conducted in the US where healthy eating awareness is higher than in the UK and has been promoted over two decades. Thus the current elderly cohorts in the US are likely to have been more exposed to the promotion of healthy eating, in particular related to control of cardiovascular diseases, than their UK counterparts and hence be more receptive to the intervention. This may further limit the generalisability of the studies to elderly people in the UK.

Recommendations

Healthy eating interventions specifically targeting elderly people need further evaluation in the UK context. These interventions should implement nutritional guidelines for this age group and include minimum nutritional requirements for elderly people as well as interventions to reduce disease risk. It is likely that interventions using group participation with goal setting offer the best way of delivering the interventions.

The elderly are a heterogeneous group and more research is required to identify and evaluate healthy eating interventions in different age groups, gender, living and socioeconomic circumstances, and by health status.

Healthy eating interventions must take account of differing nutritional requirements according to age and health status. Individual dietary assessment or a screening checklist require further exploration.

Evaluation of healthy eating interventions in elderly people requires high quality randomised controlled studies using validated measures of outcome and including both objective and subjective measures of nutrient intake, and dietary behaviour.

More attention should be paid to methods for assessing nutritional status of elderly people, for example measurement of energy expenditure.

Innovative interventions such as gardening projects, social programmes including physical activities, require further evaluation in view of their potential to enhance quality of life.

Healthy eating guidelines for elderly people should be based on appropriate evidence from epidemiological studies in elderly people on the associations between dietary intakes and disease risk. These data are particularly lacking in very elderly people.

Appendices

Appendix A. Literature search methodology

The review methodology was based on guidelines provided by the NHS Centre for Reviews and Dissemination in the publication *Undertaking systematic reviews of research on effectiveness* (CRD Report No. 4, January 1996).

Inclusion and exclusion criteria

Studies were included in the review if they met all of the following eligibility criteria:

1. *Target population:* Free living (i.e. community dwelling and not institutionalised) elderly individuals above the age of 65 years were included in this review. Studies with lower age cut-off points were also included if a substantial proportion of the participants were aged above 65. Specifically selected medical disease groups were excluded, as were individuals selected for being at raised risk of disease, for example due to elevated blood cholesterol, blood pressure, body mass or family history of disease.

2. *Research design:* Studies using experimental and quasi-experimental designs were included for review. That is, randomised controlled trials, controlled non-randomised studies and uncontrolled studies with pre- and post-intervention measures. We also included two studies with post-intervention data only.

3. *Intervention:* Any intervention designed to promote healthy eating was included. The only exception to this was interventions designed to prevent hypertension through healthy eating. These were excluded on the basis that they have been reviewed recently elsewhere (Ebrahim and Davey Smith, 1996). General health promotion packages containing a nutrition component were included for review providing there were separate data relating to the nutritional outcome(s).

4. *Outcomes:* Evaluations presenting outcomes relating to dietary behaviour or diet-related physiological measures were included in this review, as were outcomes measuring dietary knowledge, attitudes and beliefs.

5. *Geographical location/language:* Studies from developed countries were included in this review. These also had to be published in the English language.

6. *Timeframe:* Studies published between 1985 and the end of 1996 were included.

Literature searching

Published and unpublished studies were identified through a combination of systematic electronic database searching, hand searching and consultation with key organisations and experts in the field.

The database search strategy was developed and piloted on Medline. Reviews which had been identified in the preliminary search process were used at this stage to validate and refine the search strategy. The final list of terms used for the Medline search is shown in Appendix B. The Medline search strategy was then used as a model for developing search terms on other databases. The following bibliographic databases were searched:

Medline
EMBASE
SCI (Science Citation Index)
SSCI (Social Science Citation Index)
CINAHL (Cumulative Index to Nursing and Allied Health Literature)
PsychLIT
UNICORN (HEA database)
ASSIA (Applied Social Science Index and Abstracts)
SIGLE (System for Information on Grey Literature in Europe).

In total, 4 951 references were generated from these database searches. The output from each database was then coded for inclusion or exclusion (and reason for exclusion) according to the eligibility criteria. This was done in two phases. First, articles were excluded where possible on the basis of the information provided in the abstract. Where this information was insufficient the original papers were obtained in order to confirm inclusion or exclusion from the review. In particular, a large number of papers had to be checked for participant age-range and/or age-breakdown data. This second round of exclusions left only the articles to be included in the review remaining (24 articles). The results of these searches are tabulated in Appendix C.

Hand searching was conducted by checking the reference lists of identified research and review articles. Key journals in the field were also searched by hand for the last six months of 1996 (i.e. the time period not covered by the electronic databases containing these journals). The main journals searched were: *Journal of the American Dietetic Association,*

Journal of Nutrition Education, *Journal of Nutrition for the Elderly* and *Nutrition Reviews*.

A further four articles were located for inclusion in the review through hand searching, bringing the total number of articles included in the review to 28.

A list of the key organisations and individuals who responded to appeals for help in locating grey literature is given in Appendix F. An appeal for grey literature was also circulated to various electronic mailbase lists (epidemiology, public health, nutrition and evidence-based health).

Evaluation of studies

A standardised data extraction form was completed for all studies included in the review. The data extraction form, designed by the authors, includes calculations of effect size where none was given in the original paper and where sufficient information was given to carry out these calculations. Also included are details of the study design, sample size, measurement tool validity, statistical techniques, response and withdrawal rates, generalisability, feasibility, and cost effectiveness (where possible). Completed data extraction forms for each of the reviewed studies are available on request from the authors. An example of a completed data extraction form is given in Appendix E. This is in addition to the detailed summary tables provided for these studies (Appendix D).

Appendix B. Search strategy

The Medline search strategy consisted of study design terms *and* content terms *and* method terms *not* exclusion terms. Other database search terms were based on the Medline search strategy.

Study design terms

1. explode "REVIEW-LITERATURE"/all subheadings
2. REVIEW* in TI,AB,MESH
3. META-ANALY*
4. METAANALY*
5. (SYSTEMATIC*) near4 (REVIEW* or OVERVIEW*)
6. "META-ANALYSIS"
7. REVIEW in PT
8. REVIEW-ACADEMIC in PT
9. REVIEW-LITERATURE in PT
10. REVIEW-MULTICASE in PT
11. REVIEW-OF-REPORTED-CASES in PT
12. HISTORICAL-ARTICLE in PT
13. LETTER in PT
14. META-ANALYSIS in PT
15. explode "RANDOMIZED-CONTROLLED-TRIALS"/all subheadings
16. RANDOMIZED-CONTROLLED-TRIAL in PT
17. RANDOM* CONTROL* TRIAL* OR RANDOM* TRIAL*
18. RANDOM* CONTROL* STUD* OR RANDOM* STUD*
19. RANDOM* ALLOCAT*
20. RANDOM* ASSIGN*
21. explode "DOUBLE-BLIND-METHOD"/all subheadings
22. explode "SINGLE-BLIND-METHOD"/all subheadings
23. explode "RANDOM-ALLOCATION"/all subheadings
24. (SINGL* or DOUBL*) near4 (BLIND* or MASK*)
25. CONTROLLED-CLINICAL-TRIAL in PT
26. CLINICAL-TRIAL in PT
27. explode "CLINICAL-TRIALS"/all subheadings
28. explode "CONTROLLED-CLINICAL-TRIALS"/all subheadings
29. (CLIN* or CONTROL*) near4 (TRIAL* or STUD*)
30. RANDOM* in TI, AB
31. explode "RESEARCH-DESIGN"/all subheadings
32. COMPARATIVE STUD*
33. explode "EVALUATION STUDIES"/all subheadings
34. explode "PROGRAM EVALUATION"/all subheadings
35. explode "INTERVENTION STUDIES"/all subheadings
36. explode "FOLLOW-UP STUDIES"/all subheadings
37. explode "PROSPECTIVE STUDIES"/all subheadings
38. explode "COHORT-STUDIES"/all subheadings
39. explode "LONGITUDINAL-STUDIES"/all subheadings

40. explode "CASE-CONTROL-STUDIES"/all subheadings
41. "CROSS-SECTIONAL-STUDIES"
42. explode "RETROSPECTIVE-STUDIES"/all subheadings
43. explode "PILOT-PROJECTS"/all subheadings
44. explode "OUTCOME-AND-PROCESS-ASSESSMENT-(HEALTH-CARE)"/all subheadings
45. explode "NURSING-EVALUATION-RESEARCH"/all subheadings
46. (CROSS-SECTION*) near4 (TRIAL* or STUD*)
47. (COHORT) near4 (STUD* or TRIAL*)
48. (CASE-CONTROL) near4 (TRIAL* or STUD*)
49. OBSERVATION* STUD*

Content terms

1. explode "AGED"/all subheadings
2. explode "AGED,-80-AND-OVER"/all subheadings
3. explode "FRAIL-ELDERLY"/all subheadings
4. ELDERLY
5. SENIOR CITIZEN*
6. PENSIONER*
7. OLD* ADULT*
8. OLD* AGE*
9. explode "ADOLESCENCE"/all subheadings
10. explode "CHILD"/all subheadings
11. explode "CHILD,-PRESCHOOL"/all subheadings
12. explode "INFANT"/all subheadings
13. (#1 or #2 or #3 or #4 or #5 or #6 or #7 or #8)
14. (#9 or #10 or #11 or #12)
15. (#13 not #14)
16. explode "DIET"/all subheadings
17. explode "NUTRITION"/all subheadings
18. explode "NUTRITION-ASSESSMENT"/ all subheadings
19. explode "DIET-SURVEYS"/all subheadings
20. explode "NUTRITION-SURVEYS"/all subheadings
21. explode "NUTRITIONAL-STATUS"/all subheadings
22. explode "FOOD-HABITS"/all subheadings
23. explode "FOOD-PREFERENCES"/all subheadings
24. explode "DIETARY-FIBER"/all subheadings
25. explode "DIETARY-FATS"/all subheadings
26. explode "DIET,-FAT-RESTRICTED"/all subheadings
27. explode "DIET,-ATHEROGENIC"/all subheadings
28. explode "FRUIT"/ without-subheadings, supply-and-distribution
29. explode "VEGETABLES"/without-subheadings, supply-and-distribution
30. explode "BREAD"/without-subheadings, supply-and-distribution
31. explode "CEREALS"/without-subheadings, supply-and-distribution
32. NUTRITION

33. DIET
34. (NUTRITION* or DIET*) near4 (PRACTICE* or BEHAVIO* or CHANG* or EDUCAT* or PROMOT* or PROGRAM* or CAMPAIGN* or PROJECT* or ADVICE* or INTERVENTION* or COUNSEL* or COURSE* or EVALUAT* or IMPACT*)
35. HEALTH* EAT*

Method terms
1. explode "HEALTH-EDUCATION"/all subheadings
2. explode "PATIENT-EDUCATION"/all subheadings
3. "HEALTH-BEHAVIOR"/all subheadings
4. explode "PREVENTIVE-HEALTH-SERVICES"/all subheadings
5. explode "NUTRITION-POLICY"/all subheadings
6. explode "HEALTH-PLANNING"/all subheadings
7. explode "NUTRITION-SURVEYS"/all subheadings
8. explode "HEALTH-PROMOTION"/all subheadings
9. explode "TEACHING"/all subheadings
10. explode "HEALTH-PLANNING"/all subheadings
11. (EVALUAT* or EFFECT* or EFFICACY or CHANG* or RESULT* or IMPACT* or ADHERE* or SCREEN*) near4 (INITIATIVE* or INTERVENTION* or PROGRAM* or EDUCATION* or ADVICE* or COUNSEL* or PROMOT* or CAMPAIGN* or BEHAVIO* or COURSE* or PROJECT*)

Exclusion terms
1. explode "DIABETES-MELLITUS"/drug-therapy, therapy
2. explode "EATING-DISORDERS"/all subheadings
3. explode "DIABETIC-DIET"/all subheadings
4. explode "HYPERLIPIDEMIA"/drug-therapy, therapy
5. explode "OBESITY"/diet therapy, drug-therapy, therapy
6. explode "CARDIOVASCULAR-DISEASES"/drug-therapy, therapy
7. explode "NEOPLASMS"/drug-therapy, therapy
8. explode "HYPERTENSION"/drug-therapy , therapy
9. explode "HEALTH-EDUCATION,-DENTAL"/all subheadings
10. explode "DEVELOPING-COUNTRIES"/all subheadings

Appendix C. Results of database searches

Table C.1. First round exclusions

Database	Medline	SCI	SSCI	CINAHL	PsychLIT	UNICORN	EMBASE	ASSIA	SIGLE	Total
Articles found	656	769	189	456	101	149	302*	274	22	2 918*
Articles kept	79	24	2	19	11	5	28	0	0	168
Articles excluded	577	745	187	437	90	144	274	274	22	2 750
Reasons:										
Specific disease group	118	206	40	144	18	15	80	79	6	706
Wrong age-range or no age breakdown	19	122	20	6	5	2	16	78	0	268
Risk factor study	93	106	16	9	3	15	14	9	0	265
Validation study	49	5	0	5	1	6	0	0	0	66
Not dietary	145	103	32	105	6	0	8	28	1	428
Dietary, but no intervention	78	114	37	74	22	80	36	58	12	511
Dietary intervention but not health promotion	2	13	2	0	0	0	8	0	1	26
KAB survey or recommendations for health promotion	20	19	15	64	22	4	23	5	0	172
Congregate meal programmes	1	8	0	2	2	1	10	0	0	24
Other methodology	36	31	5	10	2	1	12	4	1	102
Reviews or commentaries	16	8	6	8	0	0	33	8	0	79
Duplicate publication/ already have reference	0	10	14	10	9	20	34	5	1	103

* The EMBASE database generated over 2 000 references alone – three times as many articles as any other single database search. Since it would have been too time-consuming to code all 2 335 references, the authors discarded 2 033 of the most unsuitable articles upon reading, before coding the remaining 302 (more relevant) references.

Table C.2. Second round exclusions

Database:	All databases
Articles found	168
Articles kept	24*
Articles excluded	144
Reasons:	
Specific disease group	16
Wrong age-range or no age breakdown	30
Insufficient age-breakdown data	4
Validation study	1
Not dietary	2
Dietary, but no intervention	26
Dietary intervention but not health promotion	1
Intervention, but not dietary	1
KAB survey or recommendations for health promotion	7
Congregate meal programmes	9
Other methodology	8
Reviews or commentaries	17
High blood pressure prevention	3
Supplementation	4
Abstract available only	2
Preliminary abstract subsequently superseded by a full evaluation	1
Inadequate data for review or insufficient description of outcomes	8
No outcomes – case study	1
Duplicate publication/already have reference	3

* A further four articles were located for inclusion in the review through hand searching.

Appendix D. Summary tables of reviewed studies

Table D.1. Nutrition interventions in elderly people in the community meal setting

Author	Participants	Intervention	Outcomes	Results	Reviewer's comments
		Randomised controlled trials			
Mitic, 1985	Recipients of meals programme at Salvation Army, Buffalo, New York, USA, who were classified as eating inadequately. Mainly aged 65–74. N = 66; Intervention group = 34 Control group = 32 Unit = individual.	Nutrition intervention only. *Nutrition content:* Preparation of nutritionally balanced meals. Evaluation of present eating habits. Individual nutrition goals. *Method:* Formal instruction and group participation. *Intensity:* Not stated. *Model:* Motivational. *Delivery:* No details. *Length:* 4 weeks.	24-hour dietary recall. Possible interviewer/ respondent bias. *Collection:* Not known. *Timing:* Immediately post intervention + 6 weeks post intervention.	62% of intervention and 9% of control (p < 0.05) classified as eating adequately* immediately post intervention, and 73% of intervention and 9% of control in this category 6 weeks post intervention. * At least 67% RDA for each of 8 key nutrients. *Withdrawals:* Not stated.	Large effects of intervention seen in this group with nutritional deficiencies. Limitations of self-report data. Probably generalisable in similar settings. Group participation essential component of intervention. May be resource intensive. Longer-term follow-up required.
		Experimental controlled studies			
Mayeda and Anderson, 1993	Recipients of meals programmes in Colorado, USA. Aged 60–90 years. 70% female. N = 44; 34% dropout; Intervention group =18 Control group = 11 completed the study. Unit: = site.	Multifactorial intervention: exercise and nutrition. *Nutrition content:* Lowering fat and cholesterol intake, reducing calories, making healthier food choices. Feedback on dietary records. *Method:* Postal educational package. *Intensity:* Single postal intervention. *Model:* Health beliefs. Model of acceptance of change. *Delivery:* Not stated. *Length:* 2 months.	2-day food record. Bertolli Heart Health Quiz. Nutrition Attitude Survey. *Collection:* Not known. *Timing:* 2 months post intervention.	Main outcomes not presented. Authors state no differences as control group also altered behaviour. Authors note discrepancies between self-reported behaviour and food diaries. *Withdrawals:* 35%	High default rate in both groups. Inadequate presentation of study results. Probably low cost intervention but analysis of food records and feedback may be resource intensive.

Table D.1. Nutrition interventions in elderly people in the community meal setting (contd)

		Uncontrolled experimental studies		
Author	**Participants**	**Intervention**	**Outcomes**	**Results**	**Reviewer's comments**

Author	Participants	Intervention	Outcomes	Results	Reviewer's comments
Hermann et al., 1990	Recipients of congregate meals programmes in Oklahoma, USA. Aged 60–88 years. 71% female. N = 24	Multifactorial intervention: exercise and nutrition. *Nutrition content:* Knowledge of fat, cholesterol, salt, sugar, fibre, calcium. Nutritional needs in ageing. Meeting nutritional needs through food variety. *Method:* Didactic. Verbal presentations with handouts. Training tapes. *Intensity:* One hour weekly. *Model:* Not stated. *Delivery:* Nutrition education specialist. *Length:* 12 weeks.	24-hour dietary recall. Blood pressure. Anthropometry. Cholesterol triglycerides Nutrition knowledge. *Collection:* Trained interviewers. *Timing:* immediately post intervention.	Significant changes with reduced blood pressure, triglycerides, total and LDL cholesterol (increase in HDL cholesterol). Small and largely non-significant changes in body fat and weight. Very large and significant changes in nutrition knowledge. *Withdrawals:* None stated.	Changes in lipids and blood pressure compatible with small effect (effect size 0.2), but lack of control group makes it difficult to attribute change to the intervention. Intervention feasible in most settings (walking programme may be more problematic).

Table D.2. Nutrition interventions in elderly people in communal settings (contd)

		Randomised controlled trials		
Author	**Participants**	**Intervention**	**Outcomes**	**Results**	**Reviewer's comments**

Author	**Participants**	**Intervention**	**Outcomes**	**Results**	**Reviewer's comments**
Bedell and Shackleton, 1989	Attending community centre in housing project in New York City, USA. Aged 60–88 years. 86% female. 83% white. $N = 29$; Intervention group = 15 Control group = 14 Unit = individual.	Nutrition intervention only. *Nutrition content:* Basic 4 food groups. Nutrients. Food and ageing. Consumer issues. *Method:* Didactic. Classes and handouts. *Intensity:* 4 one-hour classes. *Model:* Educational: goal setting. *Delivery:* 2 nurses. *Length:* 2 weeks.	24-hour dietary recall. Nutrition knowledge. Interviewers not stated (researchers?) – possible interviewer bias. *Collection:* Interviewers. *Timing:* Immediately post intervention.	No significant differences observed between the groups in summary scores for nutrition knowledge and 24-hour diet recall. *Withdrawals:* None.	Possible study contamination as controls attended same centre. Study underpowered to detect between-group differences in knowledge of a moderate effect, but minimal change in dietary behaviour observed. Interpretation of summary score for 24-hour recall problematic. Feasible intervention for other settings. Longer-term outcomes needed.
Kupka-Schutt and Mitchell, 1992	Members of a local hospital Seniors Program in Washington State, USA. 70% aged 65–74. 70% female. $N = 125$; Intervention group = 35 Control group A = 32 Control group B = 58 Unit = individual.	Nutrition intervention only. *Nutrition content:* Evaluation of food intake, instruction on needs and nutrient intake of group. Setting of individual dietary goals. *Method:* Facilitator-led groups. *Intensity:* 4 one-hour sessions. *Model:* Motivational (Mitic's Nutrition Instruction Model). *Delivery:* Nutritionist *Length:* Not stated. Control A: 4 lectures on dietary guidelines.	3-day food records. DIF scores, % RDAs. *Collection:* Postal following instruction at baseline. *Timing:* 2 months post intervention.	No significant differences between groups in DIF scores (dietary quality) but no data presented. Significant within intervention group improvements in proportion eating less than RDAs for dairy products and bread. Both intervention and control A showed significant decreases in fat compared with control B. *Withdrawals:* 36% from control group B.	Poor presentation of results and statistical tests. Bias due to high withdrawals in control group B. Although the intervention group improved RDAs more than the other groups, fat reduction was of a similar order in the group receiving the simple instruction sessions. This group also had a more favourable trend in other nutrients.

Table D.2. Nutrition interventions in elderly people in communal settings (contd)

Author	Participants	Intervention	Outcomes	Results	Reviewer's comments
		Randomised controlled trials			
Haber and Lacy, 1993	Attenders at a multidisciplinary geriatric centre in a mid-west metropolitan area in the US. Aged 55–94 years. Mean age 68 years. 75% white. N = 57; Intervention group =29 Control group = 28 Unit = individual.	Multifactorial intervention: exercise, stress management and nutrition. *Nutrition content:* Not described. *Method:* Didactic in both intervention in control + in intervention group, peer support with individual contracts and physician wellness prescriptions. *Intensity:* Not stated. *Model:* Behavioural contracting. *Delivery:* Multidisciplinary team of health professionals. Nurse facilitated peer group sessions. *Length:* 10 weeks.	*Nutrition:* Eating habits. *Others:* Stress management, functional status. *Collection:* Interview administered. *Timing:* Immediately post intervention.	Significantly more people in the intervention group reported increasing fibre intake (4-fold) and reducing sodium (3-fold). *Withdrawals:* 11% overall.	Study underpowered to detect other than large effects. Intervention group received personal physician wellness prescriptions as well as peer educators and the relative effects cannot be separated. Resource intensive.
		Experimental controlled studies			
Higgins, 1988 Higgins, 1989	Living in senior citizen housing units in Albuquerque, New Mexico, USA. Mean age 76 years. N = 91; Intervention = 34 Control group 1 = 33 Control group 2 = 24 (Control group 2 drawn from elderly attending exercise class). Unit = site.	Multifactorial intervention: medical self-care activities, nutrition, fitness and relaxation. *Nutrition content:* Basic 4 foods and water. Nutrition density. 24-hour recall: starch, protein and fibre. *Method:* Workshop and activity sessions. Didactic. *Intensity:* 4 workshop sessions of 2.5 hr and 4 activity sessions of 2 hours. *Model:* Self-responsibility. *Delivery:* Nurse. *Length:* 1 month.	*Biometric:* BP, total and HDL cholesterol. Anthropometry. Flexibility. Collected by 'blinded' observers for intervention and control groups. *Health behaviours:* Standard questionnaires. *Collection:* Not stated. *Timing:* 6 weeks post intervention.	Significant within-group changes for intervention group for decreased cholesterol (−10% compared with control) and increased HDL cholesterol (+20% compared with control) and % body fat. Behavioural questionnaire found statistically significant between-group difference in favour of intervention for most eating behaviours. *Withdrawals:* None.	Well conducted study with objective outcome data collected by observers blind to intervention group. Statistical analysis failed to test the between-group changes in biometric outcomes and to take account of cluster allocation. Apparent effects on cholesterol were large. Longer-term outcomes required. Study seems feasible in a communal setting.

Table D.2. Nutrition interventions in elderly people in communal settings (contd)

		Experimental controlled studies			
Author	Participants	Intervention	Outcomes	Results	Reviewer's comments
Dennison *et al.*, 1991 Dennison *et al.*, 1992	Living in subsidised housing sites for elderly, New York, USA. Mean age 76 years. 90% female. 90% + white. *N* = 93; Intervention A = 40 Intervention B = 43 Cortrol = 10 Unit = site.	Nutrition intervention only. *Nutrition content:* Basic nutrition. Individual diet analysis and goals (Groups A and B). *Method:* Group A – interactive computer program for diet analysis, in addition to didactic methods (Group B). *Intensity:* 4 one-hour classes. *Model:* 'Hands-on' activated learning. *Delivery:* Dietitians. *Length:* 4 weeks.	3-day food records. Satisfaction with programme. *Collection:* Self-completed. *Timing:* 1 week post intervention.	Significant differences in favour of *both* interventions compared to control in declines in saturated fat, and similar trend for monosaturated fats. No other dietary results reported. No differences between the intervention groups in the programme satisfaction questionnaires. *Withdrawals:* Not stated.	Nutrition outcome data not available for 75% of both intervention groups. No information on number *originally* in control group. Serious concerns about possible bias due to missing data and loss of study power. Possible large effects of intervention on fat intake. Results must be treated with extreme caution.
Rose, 1992	Living in senior citizens' independent housing unit in the USA. Mean age 75 years. 85% female. 67% black. *N* = 155; Intervention = 61 Control = 94 Unit = site.	Peer educators (*n* = 13) at intervention sites trained in multifactorial intervention including nutrition. *Nutrition content:* Low fat diets. *Method:* Information on peer educators disseminated in residents' newsletter. *Intensity:* 8 two-hour sessions. *Model:* Social Learning Theory. *Delivery:* Not stated. *Length:* 4 months.	Dietary knowledge and behaviour. Heart disease risk factors. *Collection:* Interviewer. *Timing:* 3 months after training of peer educators.	Significant between group differences favouring intervention for self-reported fat intake and knowledge of heart disease risk factors. *Withdrawals:* Only one-third in control and intervention participation in survey. Further 11% of those with baseline had no follow-up data.	Unusual study design involving training of peer educators and an informal intervention delivery. Only one-third of residents in both control and intervention participated in survey. Possible substantial selection bias.

Table D.2. Nutrition interventions in elderly people in communal settings (contd)

Experimental controlled studies

Author	Participants	Intervention	Outcomes	Results	Reviewer's comments
Constans *et al.*, 1994	Students from the University of the Third Age in Tours, France. Average age 68 years. 55% female. *N* = 123; Assigned to intervention and control groups on the basis of entry calcium levels. Unit = individual.	Nutrition intervention only. *Nutrition content:* Focus to increase dietary calcium intake. *Method:* Dietary advice and feedback on 7-day food record. *Intensity:* Not stated. *Model:* Not stated. *Delivery:* Dietitian. *Length:* One-off advice.	7-day food diaries. *Collection:* Self-completed. *Timing:* 2 years post intervention.	Significant increases in dietary calcium in intervention group. *Withdrawals:* 56% with no outcome data.	Those with low calcium intakes at entry showed significant and large improvements after 2 years but an appropriate control group was not used and these changes could in part be explained by regression to the mean. There was a high number of withdrawals.

Uncontrolled experimental studies

Author	Participants	Intervention	Outcomes	Results	Reviewer's comments
Goldberg *et al.*, 1989	Local chapters of the American Association of Retired Persons in Massachusetts, USA. Aged 55–89 years. 78% female. *N* = 244.	Nutrition intervention only. *Nutrition content:* Focused on weight control, food safety, dietary sodium, nutritional supplements. *Method:* 'TV' quiz game shown to participants. *Intensity:* One 27-minute video. *Model:* Not stated. *Delivery:* By video to local chapter meetings. *Length:* One-off $1\frac{1}{2}$-hour show.	Nutrition knowledge. *Collection:* self-administered questionnaire. *Timing:* Immediately prior to and post intervention; and mailed 4 months post intervention.	Large improvement immediately after show in knowledge (59% correct prior to show v. 84% correct post show). This declined to 72% correct at 4 months post intervention. Total number of participants not known – only those who completed questionnaires. *Withdrawals:* 6% did not complete immediate post-test questionnaire. Response to 4 months post test not given.	Possible Hawthorne effect of knowledge of participants in evaluation on immediate recall. Videotape of quiz show shown in communal setting not equivalent to TV show. Costs of intervention not addressed, but likely to be considerable (included well-known comedian).

Table D.2. Nutrition interventions in elderly people in communal settings (contd)

	Uncontrolled experimental studies			
Author	**Participants**	**Intervention**	**Outcomes**	**Results**	**Reviewer's comments**
Doshi *et al.*, 1994	Volunteers to programme conducted in local church in Akron, Ohio, USA. Aged 55–86 years. Average 72 years. 87% female. 100% African-American. N = 31.	Multifactorial intervention: nutrition and fitness. *Nutrition content:* Energy, fats, cholesterol and sodium. Cookery demonstrations to reduce fat and cholesterol. *Method:* Didactic with physical activities. *Intensity:* Biweekly; duration not given. *Model:* Not stated. *Delivery:* Staff not stated. *Length:* 10 weeks.	Glucose, cholesterol and triglycerides. Diet history and 24-hour recall. Anthropometry. Exercise history. *Collection:* Dietary data collected by student interviewers. *Timing:* Immediately post intervention.	Significant reductions in total and LDL cholesterol. No significant differences in dietary intakes of calories, protein, fats or carbohydrates. Waist circumference significantly decreased. *Withdrawals:* Not stated.	Potential for bias in collection of dietary and anthropometric data. Significant decreases in lipids of a small magnitude but lack of control group weakens evidence for intervention.

Table D.3. Nutrition interventions in the elderly population living in the community

		Experimental controlled studies			
Author	**Participants**	**Intervention**	**Outcomes**	**Results**	**Reviewer's comments**
Egger et al., 1991	Residents aged 55+ in 3 small communities (2 intervention: 1 control) with a high proportion of retired people in New South Wales, Australia. 650–850 residents in each community. Unit = community.	Nutrition intervention only. Nutrition content: Information on bread and its benefits. Method: (1)Community strategy – media, pricing, social marketing versus (2) patient education – pamphlets handed out by local doctors. Intensity: Not stated. Model: Not stated. Delivery: As above. Length: 4 months.	Wholemeal/wholegrain bread sales. Laxative sales. Collection: Weekly sales information from local bakeries and pharmacists. Timing: 2 weeks post intervention.	50% increase in bread sales and similar decreases in laxative sales in community strategy compared to either patient education or control.	Large effect of community intervention campaign but costs and resources to mount this campaign are not described.
Crockett et al., 1992	Randomly selected from drivers' icence lists in N. Dakota, USA. Aged 60–70 years. 61% female. 85% participation. N = 399 at baseline; Full intervention = 146 Minimum intervention = 87 Control = 102 Unit = community.	Nutrition intervention only. Nutrition content: All intervention subjects received 3 newsletters with information on dietary fat, fibre and healthy food purchasing. Full intervention also received additional incentives – shopping coupons, free cholesterol tests, etc. Method: Information packs. Intensity: 3 newsletters mailed at 2-week intervals. Model: Not stated. Delivery: Postal and in full intervention telephone follow-up. Length: 6 weeks.	Dietary knowledge. Shelf inventory. Food frequency questionnaire. Collection: By post. Timing: 6 weeks post intervention.	No significant differences between control and intervention groups for any outcomes. Data presented only for those with pre- and post-intervention questionnaires (84% of sample). Results for dietary knowledge and shelf inventory stated as not statistically significant, but no results shown. Withdrawals: 16% with no post-intervention data. Breakdown by group not known.	Numbers of subjects per group at baseline not shown. Random sampling and high response rate probably ensure representative sample. Low-cost mailed intervention but free cholesterol testing and food coupons might entail considerable cost in the mass setting.

Table D.3. Nutrition interventions in the elderly population living in the community (contd)

			Uncontrolled experimental studies		
Author	**Participants**	**Intervention**	**Outcomes**	**Results**	**Reviewer's comments**
Weiss and Davis, 1985	Systematic sample of households receiving a community newspaper for seniors in S. Kansas, USA. Median age group 60–69 years. 81% female *N* = 326.	Nutrition intervention only. *Nutrition content:* Topic-related: covered fibre, sodium, food and drug interactions, saving nutrients in food. Recipes based on high fibre, low fat, low sodium. Interviews with elderly peer recipe testers. *Method:* Print media. *Intensity:* Monthly. *Model:* Not stated. *Delivery:* Monthly article in free seniors' newsletter. *Length:* 11 months.	24-item questionnaire on cooking habits, nutrition information and behavioural changes. *Collection:* Telephone interview. *Timing:* End of 5 articles.	Descriptive post-intervention results. 91% response rate. Two-thirds reported reading articles. 17% reported changes in diet (increased fibre, reduced salt).	Descriptive data only. Sample limited to telephone subscribers and biased towards high-income elderly. Self-reported behavioural change in less than one in five of readership. Feasibility in other settings dependent on newspaper targeted at elderly and required costs and resources.
Hackman and Wagner, 1990	Home owners in Oregon and Pennsylvania, USA (3 sites). Mean age 68 years. 70% female. 72% white. *N* = 108.	Nutrition and gardening intervention. *Nutrition content:* 7 nutritional areas for improvement sources of vitamins, iron, fibre and dairy products. *Method:* Didactic and printed materials + provision of gardening boxes and instruction. *Intensity:* Bimonthly sessions and home visits. *Model:* Perception of control and social support. *Delivery:* Nutritionists, dietitians, master gardeners. *Length:* 5 months.	Food frequency questionnaires. Attitudinal scales. *Collection:* Interviewer administered. *Timing:* Not stated.	Analysed by site. Oregon site showed greatest improvements for most of the 7 nutrients while low-income urban sites showed increased consumption only for dairy products and water and a possible decrease in some nutrients. *Withdrawals:* No withdrawals but post-intervention dietary data missing in one-third at one site.	Innovative approach to nutrition education through provision of garden boxes and garden lessons in addition to traditional nutrition education. Greatest benefits in the oiginal demonstration site but less convincing in the low-income areas. Intensive in resources.

Table D.3. Nutrition interventions in the elderly population living in the community (contd)

	Experimental controlled studies			
Author	**Participants**	**Intervention**	**Outcomes**	**Results**	**Reviewer's comments**
Lach, Dwyer and Mann, 1994	10% systematic sample for post-intervention evaluation, in 3 major cities in USA covering nearly 10 000 recipients of intervention materials. Mean age 72 years. 81% female. N = 348.	Nutrition intervention only. *Nutrition content:* Low fat, high fibre, low sodium, high calcium. Principles of food nutrition for older adults. *Method:* Booklets. *Intensity:* Variable. *Model:* Not stated. *Delivery:* Stall in supermarkets, community centres and hospitals. Volunteer staff. *Length:* Up to 2 weeks.	24-hour recall of food types. Questions on changes in dietary habits. *Collection:* Postal. *Timing:* 4–8 weeks post intervention.	Descriptive post-intervention results. 35% response rate. 58% reported making changes as a result of programme.	Descriptive data only. Low response rate makes results of doubtful validity and generalisability. Large programme targeted at over 10 000 adults and involving large resources of staff and commitment.
	Cross-sectional survey				
Butler, Ohls and Posner, 1985	Random sample from 6 sites of people aged over 65 years and eligible for Food Stamp Program (FSP). N = 1584 (no breakdown by participants/non-participants).	Nutrition intervention only. Stamps (or money equivalents) provided to low-income households for use in food stores. FSP introduced in 1979.	*Dietary:* 24-hour recall. *Collection:* Interviewer administered.	Very small differences in nutrient intake between participants and non-participants. Only calcium intake significantly increased.	No data on response rates of FSP participants/non-participants. No estimates of study precision. Multiple regression analyses used to control for possible confounding but substantial bias may remain in a non-randomised evaluation.

Table D.4. Nutrition interventions as part of health promotion interventions

			Randomised controlled trials		
Author	**Participants**	**Intervention**	**Outcomes**	**Results**	**Reviewer's comments**
Leigh et al., 1992 Fries et al., 1993	Retired Bank of America employees in California, USA. Average age 68 years. 52% female. N = 4013; Intervention = 1089 Control group 1 = 1017 Control group 2 = 1907 Unit = club.	Multifactorial Health Trac Program: diet, exercise, smoking, alcohol. *Nutrition content:* Personal computerised feedback to lifestyle questionnaires. *Method:* Postal. *Intensity:* 6 monthly. *Model:* Self-sufficiency. *Delivery:* Postal. *Length:* 6 monthly with evaluation at 1 and 2 years. Control group 1 switched to intervention at 1 year.	Lifestyle questionnaires. Self-reported cholesterol and weight. Same questionnaires as used for intervention (not available for control group 2). Claims data from medical insurance records – available by group for all groups. *Collection:* Postal. *Timing:* 6 months.	Significant differences favouring intervention in self-reported dietary habits. Largest differences (around 10%) for reduced fat, salt, dairy products, and increase in wholegrain breads. No differences in self-reported cholesterol or weight. *Withdrawals:* 16% in both groups by year 1.	Large trial providing precise estimates of effect with favourable dietary trends in the intervention group. Analyses not adjusted for cluster randomisation in multiple testing. No objective outcomes. Economic analyses are of questionable validity. Good compliance with programme with nearly 80% still participating after 2 years.
Ives, Kuller and Traven, 1993 Lave et al., 1996	Medicare beneficiaries in rural Pennsylvania, USA. Aged 65–79 years. Mean age 71 years. 57% female. Mainly white. N = 3884; Capitation = 1312 Fee for service = 1347 Control = 1225 Unit = individual.	Multifactorial: nutrition, smoking cessation, alcohol counselling, influenza immunisation. *Nutrition content:* 41% in the 2 intervention groups eligible for cholesterol lowering (25%) or weight reduction (25%) programme. No systematic protocol – usual practice. *Method:* Individual counselling. *Intensity:* Up to 5 visits following a positive screen. *Model:* Not stated. *Delivery:* Family physicians, hospital staff (physicians, dietitians, nutritionists). *Length:* Variable.	*Group eligible for nutrition:* Blood cholesterol, use of lipid lowering drugs, attitude to cholesterol control. *All intervention subjects:* Mortality, hospitalisation, rates for CVD and pneumonia. Use of other health-care services. *Collection:* Telephone interviews, blood samples, Medicare databases. *Timing:* 2–3 years post baseline.	*Group eligible for nutrition:* Similar falls in cholesterol occurred in both intervention groups and control. Similar use of lipid lowering drugs in all groups. *All subjects:* No differences in mortality and morbidity. *Withdrawals:* Only 50% of those eligible attended for nutritional counselling. Around 25% in each group did not provide a follow-up blood sample.	Less than half of those eligible used the nutrition counselling with a slightly higher uptake in the fee for service group. No specific guidelines for cholesterol management. Both these factors might have accounted for low impact of intervention, but similar falls in cholesterol found in participants and non-participants.

Table D.4. Nutrition interventions as part of health promotion interventions (contd)

Randomised controlled trials

Author	Participants	Intervention	Outcomes	Results	Reviewer's comments
Fries et al., 1994	Employees and retired workforce receiving Blue Shield insurance in California, USA. Grouped by employees, seniors (average age 73) and retirees (average age 63). N = 35000 (retirees and seniors): Intervention = 33700 Control = 1647 Unit = individual.	Multifactorial Health Trac Program: diet, exercise, smoking, alcohol. Nutrition content: Personal computerised feedback to lifestyle questionnaires. Method: Postal. Intensity: 6 monthly. Model: Not stated. Delivery: Postal. Length: 6 monthly with evaluation at 1 and 2 years. Control group 1 switched to intervention at 1 year.	Lifestyle questionnaires only for intervention group. Claims data from medical insurance data available at individual level. Collection: Postal. Timing: 6 months.	Within-group 18 month changes from baseline showed 20% reductions in self-reported dietary fat and saturated fat. Trend to reduced costs in intervention group compared to control group. Withdrawals: Around 20% over 18 months.	Only 30% of intervention group participated. No control data available for dietary outcomes. Some unusual results in the claims analysis suggest allocation bias. Good compliance with 80% of active participants still participating after18 months.
Mayer et al., 1994 Elder et al., 1995	Medicare beneficiaries in San Diego, USA. Mean age 73 years. 56% female. 96% white. N = 1800; Intervention = 899 Control = 901 Unit = individual.	Multifactorial intervention: clinical tests and immunisation, health risk appraisal based on hierarchy of goals and choice of single goal only. Nutrition content: For hypertensives, weight loss and sodium reduction. For non-hypertensives, choice of nutrition management as the goal, and one of the following: dietary fat reduction, sodium education, fibre and cruciferous vegetable increase. Also 4 group sessions on exercise and nutrition. Method: Individual counselling and goal setting. Intensity:15-minute face-to-face counselling and 8 two-hour group sessions. Model: Kanfer's model of self-control. Delivery: Public health students. Length: 8 weeks.	215 item lifestyle questionnaire with unspecified number of nutrition items. Body Mass Index. Physical activity. Collection: Not stated. Timing:1 and 2 years post intervention.	25% chose one of the nutrition goals. Significant between group decreases in fat intake favouring intervention (compatible with effect size of 0.12). Most effects of intervention in physical activity chosen by 40%. Two-year outcomes continued to show benefits in self-reported exercise activities, but not in any dietary variables. Withdrawals: 16% from the intervention group and 12% from the control group withdrew in the first year. Over half in both groups withdrew by the end of the 2nd year.	Limitation of study design was that participants were allowed only one goal to be chosen from a hierarchy. Reduced ability of study to test benefit of nutrition component. The result for fat intake was encouraging given that only 8% chose this goal. Poor compliance with program after 2 years with only 50% still participating.

Table D.4. Nutrition interventions as part of health promotion interventions (contd)

		Prospective cohort study with historical controls			
Author	**Participants**	**Intervention**	**Outcomes**	**Results**	**Reviewer's comments**
Fries *et al.*, 1992	Blue Cross/Blue Shield beneficiaries in California, USA. 135000 aged less than 65 years and 130000 aged either 65 years or over enrolled 1986–1991 of which: 36000 aged 65– with 12-month follow-up data and 27000 with 18-month follow-up.	Multifactorial Health Trac and Senior Health Trac Program: diet, exercise, smoking, alcohol. *Nutrition content:* Personal computerised feedback to lifestyle questionnaires. *Method:* Postal. *Intensity:* 6 monthly. *Model:* Not stated. *Delivery:* Postal. *Length:* 6 monthly with evaluation at 1 and 2 years. Control group 1 switched to intervention at 1 year.	Health risk scores. Individual health risk items. Self-reported cholesterol. *Collection:* Postal. *Timing:* 6 monthly.	Similar changes observed for both under 65 and over 65 groups. From baseline 12 and 18 months large falls in self-reported intakes of 'high' dietary fat and 'high' salt intake. Very small changes in cholesterol or overweight. *Withdrawals:* 37% recently enrolled; 25% dropped out or changed insurance.	No objective measures of dietary behaviour. Self-reported cholesterol levels only available in 25%. Secular changes controlled for by concurrent baselines over 30 months of follow-up.

Appendix E. Data extraction forms for reviewed studies

Completed data extraction forms for each of the reviewed studies are available from the authors. An example of a completed data extraction form is given below.

Data extraction form

Publication information
Authors: Mitic W
Article title: Nutrition education for older adults: implementation of a nutrition instruction program
Source: Health Education 1985; Feb/March: 7–9
Country of origin: Canada
Institutional affiliation: Health Education Division, Dalhouse University, Halifax

Study classification
Study design: Randomised controlled study
Unit of allocation: Individual
Method of allocation: Random (details not given)
Target population: *Age:* Elderly
                      Sex: Both
                      Nature: High risk for poor nutrition
Setting: Congregate meals programmes setting
Geographical location: Urban and rural

Study details
Study subjects: *Age:* Aged 65+, majority aged 65–74
                      Sex: No details
                      Nature: High risk of poor nutrition. Classified at baseline as having < 67% of RDAs for any one of 8 nutrients
                      Socioeconomic group/income: Not stated but recipients of meals programme at Salvation Army
                      Ethnicity: Not stated
                      Geographical location: Buffalo, New York, USA
                      Size: Intervention group(s): 34
                      Control group: 32
                      Sample size calculation: No mention
                      Representativeness: Volunteer study. Inadequate information on sample characteristics
Intervention category: Education
Brief description of intervention: The study used a motivational model consisting of three phases. In Phase I participants were taught how to evaluate present eating habits by classification into the Four Food

Groups, followed by instruction in preparation of nutritionally balanced meals. Phase II used a cognitive framework to increase awareness of nutrition and health and economical shopping advice. These sessions used a mixture of didactic presentations and group discussions. Handouts were provided. Phase III, affective instruction, used student-centred activities to promote formulation of individual nutrition related goals.

Theoretical model: Activated Health Education Model

Timescale: Length of study: 4 weeks intervention; outcome data collected immediately post intervention (post-test1) and after a further 6 weeks (post-test 2).

Frequency of intervention: Not stated

Delivery of intervention: Staff: Not stated

Collection of outcome data: 24-hour dietary recalls administered but no description of who the interviewers were or whether they were blind to the randomised groups.

Outcome(s)	Method of assessing outcome	Validity of measurement tool
Dietary	24-hr recall for classification into 8 essential nutrients: protein, calcium, iron, vitamin A, thiamin, riboflavin, niacin, vitamin C.	Informal and simple data on validity and reliability obtained in non-study subjects.

Analysis

Statistical techniques used: Chi squared tests for changes in proportions eating at least 67% RD

A. Descriptive data only presented for individual nutrients.

Adjustment for confounding: No

Approach to analysis: Not given

Follow-up of withdrawals (and inclusion in analysis)?: Apparently no withdrawals

Results

Response rate: Not stated

Compliance with protocol: Not stated

Overall number of withdrawals: None

Outcome: Overall proportion classified as 'eating adequately' defined as taking at least 67% RDA for each of the 8 nutrients.

Statistical significance: At post-test1, 62% of intervention group compared with 9% of the control group were classified as eating adequately, $p < 0.05$, and at post test2 73% of the intervention group compared with 9% of the control group, $p < 0.05$.

Estimates of effect size: Not calculated

95% confidence intervals: Not given

Author's conclusions on effectiveness of intervention

The results of this investigation demonstrated that the nutrition education programme (NIM) based on the principles of activated health education was effective in modifying the dietary habits of the elderly in a positive healthy direction. Testing of the hypotheses revealed that the programme was not only effective in modifying, to a significant degree, their dietary habits immediately after the programme but also in sustaining this effect for six weeks after the programme had been completed.

Reviewer's conclusions on effectiveness of intervention

This study used a randomised controlled trial design to evaluate the benefits of a motivational education model to improve dietary intakes of elderly people identified as having inadequate intakes in the congregate meals programme setting. The possibility of interviewer and responder bias cannot be discounted. The intervention led to large improvements in the proportion classified as having adequate dietary intakes compared to minor improvements in the control group. These differences were sustained at the 6-week follow-up. The intervention appeared quite resource-intensive but insufficient information is provided to fully assess this. It is probably feasible within the congregate, meals programme setting or other settings where elderly people congregate, as group participation was an essential component of the intervention. The results are likely to be generalisable in similar settings to elderly people at risk of nutritional deficiency.

Overall judgement

Quality of paper:
Appropriate information included to enable judgements? Yes
Quality of study:
Replicability of design/intervention: Used structured health education model to deliver intervention
Generalisability of findings: Probably to participants within the congregate meals programme setting or similar low-income settings who have poor nutrition.
Specific reservations: Possibility of interviewer and respondent bias in the 24-hour dietary recall data.
Intervention evaluation: No data on precision or magnitude of effects given.
Practicality/feasibility of intervention: Depends on the resources required (skills, number of personnel and staff hours).

Appendix F. Organisations and individuals who responded to requests for help

Age Concern England

British Geriatrics Association

Caroline Walker Trust

Centre for Evaluation of Health Promotion and Social Interventions

Community Health

Health Promotion Information Centre, Health Education Authority

National Food Alliance

Nutrition Advisory Group for the Elderly, British Dietetic Association

Nutrition Screening Initiative, Washington DC, USA

Research into Ageing

Lorraine Ashton, Ageing Well Initiative

Prof. Robert Beaglehole, University of Auckland, New Zealand

Dr Sheila Bingham, MRC Dunn Nutrition Unit, Cambridge

Sheila Bodey, Mancunian Community Health NHS Trust

John Boyce, Pilton Community Health Project, Edinburgh, Scotland

Carolyn Bunney, Central Coast Area Health Service, Australia

Jennifer Copeland, Nutrition Advisory Group for the Elderly

Anne Donelan, Nutrition Advisory Group for the Elderly

Phyllis Eaton, Nutrition Advisory Group for the Elderly

Dr Edward Dickinson, Cochrane Field of Health Care of Older People

Dr Joyce Hughes, Nutrition Unit, Department of Health

Francis Hunt, Ageing Well Initiative

Janet Jackson, Nutrition Education Programme, Wood End, Coventry

Dr Donald Kemper, Healthwise, Idaho, USA

Prof. Kay Tee Khaw, Addenbrooke's Hospital, Cambridge

Jacqui McGinely, Castlemilk Food Co-op Development Project, Glasgow, Scotland

Dr Linda McKie, University of Aberdeen, Scotland

Dr John McKinlay, New England Research Institute, USA

Elizabeth Mills, Research into Ageing

Dr Meredith Minkler, University of California, USA

Dr Donald Patrick, University of Washington, USA

Vivien Prendiville, South Cumbria Health Promotion Unit

Ruth Rollin, Healthy Village Project, Brockenhurst

Prof. Marianne Schroll, Copenhagen City Hospital, Denmark

An appeal for grey literature was also circulated to the following electronic mailbase lists:

public-health@mailbase.ac.uk
evidence-based-health@mailbase.ac.uk
food-for-thought@mailbase.ac.uk
epidemio-l@cc.umontreal.ca
nutepi@tubvm.cs.tu-berlin.de

References

Bedell, B A and Shackleton, P A (1989). The relationship between a nutrition education program and nutrition knowledge and eating behaviors of the elderly. *Journal of Nutrition for the Elderly* **8**:35–45.

Bunney, C and Bartl, R (1996). *Reduce the risk: a common sense guide to preventing poor nutrition in older people.* Gosford, New South Wales: Nutrition Department, Central Coast Area Health Service (PO Box 361, Gosford, NSW 2250).

Butler, J S, Ohls, J C and Posner, B (1985). The effect of the food stamp program on the nutrient intake of the eligible elderly. *Journal of Human Resources* **20**:405–20.

Constans, T, Delarue, J, Rivol, M, Theret, V and Lamisse, F (1994). Effects of nutrition education on calcium intake in the elderly. *Journal of the American Dietetic Association* **94**(4):447–8.

Contento *et al.*(1995). Chapter 7: Nutrition education for older adults. *Journal of Nutrition Education* **27**(6):339–46.

Crockett, S J, Heller, K E, Skauge, L H and Merkel, J M (1992). Mailed-home nutrition education for rural seniors: a pilot study. *Journal of Nutrition Education* **24**:312–15.

Davies, L (1991). *Opportunities for better health in the elderly through mass catering: report on a study.* Copenhagen: WHO.

Dennison, K F, Dennison, D and Ward, J Y (1991). Computerized nutrition program – effect on nutrient intake of senior-citizens. *Journal of the American Dietetic Association* **91**:1431–3.

Dennison, D, Dennison, K F, Ward, J Y and Wu, Y W (1992). Satisfaction of senior citizens in a nutrition education program with and without computer-assisted instruction. *Journal of Nutrition for the Elderly* **12**(1):15–31.

Department of Health (1992a). *The health of elderly people: an epidemiological overview.* London: HMSO.

Department of Health (1992b). *The nutrition of elderly people.* Report of the Working Group on the Nutrition of Elderly People of the Committee on Medical Aspects of Food Policy. Report on Health and Social Subjects, No. 43. London: HMSO.

Doshi, N J, Hurley, R S, Garrison, M E, Stombaugh, I S, Rebovich, E J, Wodarski, L A and Farris, L (1994). Effectiveness of a nutrition education and physical fitness training program in lowering lipid levels in the black elderly. *Journal of Nutrition for the Elderly* **13**(3):23–33.

Ebrahim, S and Davey Smith, G (1996). *Health promotion in older people for the prevention of coronary heart disease and stroke.* Health Promotion Effectiveness Reviews. London: Health Education Authority.

Egger, G, Wolfenden, K, Pares, J and Mowbray, G (1991). Bread – its a great way to go – increasing bread consumption decreases laxative sales in an elderly community. *Medical Journal of Australia* **155**:820–1.

Elder, J P, Williams, S J, Drew, J A, Wright, B L, and Boulan, T E (1995). Longitudinal effects of preventive services on health behaviors among an elderly cohort. *American Journal of Preventive Medicine* **11**:354–9.

Euronut SENECA investigators (1991). Intake of vitamins and minerals. *European Journal of Clinical Nutrition* **45**: Suppl 3:121–38.

Frank, E, Winkleby, M A, Fortmann, S P and Rockhill, B (1992). Improved cholesterol-related knowledge and behavior and plasma cholesterol levels in adults during the 1980s. *Journal of the American Medical Association* September(23/30):1566–72.

Finch S, Doyle W, Lowe C, Bates C J, Prentice A, Smithers G and Clarke, P C (1997). *National Diet and Nutrition Survey: people aged 65 years or over.* Volume 1: Report of the diet and nutrition survey. London: Stationery Office.

Fries, J F, Bloch, D A, Harrington, H, Richardson, N and Beck, R (1993). Two-year results of a randomized controlled trial of a health promotion program in a retiree population: the Bank of America Study. *American Journal of Medicine* **94**(5):455–62.

Fries, J F, Fries, S T, Parcell, C L and Harrington, H (1992). Health risk changes with a low-cost individualized health promotion program: effects at up to 30 months. *American Journal of Health Promotion* **6**(5):364–71.

Fries, J F, Harrington, H, Edwards, R, Kent, L A and Richardson, N (1994). Randomized controlled trial of cost reductions from a health education program: the California public employees' retirement system (PERS) study. *American Journal of Health Promotion* **8**:216–23.

Gans, K M, Lapane, K L, Lasater, T M and Carleton, R A (1994). Effects of intervention on compliance to referral and lifestyle recommendations given at cholesterol screening programs. *American Journal of Preventive Medicine* **10**:275–82.

German, P S, Burton, L C, Shapiro, S, Steinwachs, D M, Tsuji, I, Paglia, M J and Damiano, A M (1995). Extended coverage for preventive services for the elderly: response and results in a demonstration population. *American Journal of Public Health* **85**(3):379–86.

Goldberg, J P, Gershoff, S N, Gandy, R B and Hartz, S C (1989). The effectiveness of a television quiz show in providing nutrition information to the elderly. *Journal of Nutrition for the Elderly* **21**:86–9.

Haber, D and Lacy, M G (1993). Evaluation of a socio-behavioral intervention for changing health behaviors of older adults. *Behavior, Health, & Aging* **3**(2):73–85.

Hackman, R R M and Wagner, E L (1990). The senior gardening and nutrition project: development and transport of a dietary behavior change and health promotion program. *Journal of Nutrition Education* **22**:262–70.

Hall, N, de Beck, P, Johnson, D and Mackinnon, K (1992). Randomized trial of a health promotion program for frail elders. *Canadian Journal on Aging* **11**(1):72–91.

Hermann, J R, Kopel, B H, McCrory, M L and Kulling, F A (1990). Effect of a cooperative extension nutrition and exercise program for older adults on nutrition knowledge, dietary intake, anthropometric measurements, and serum lipids. *Journal of Nutrition Education* **22**(6):271–4.

Higgins, P G (1988). Biometric outcomes of a geriatric health promotion programme. *Journal of Advanced Nursing* **13**(6):710–15.

Higgins, P G (1989). Short-term changes in health behaviours of older adults. *Canadian Journal of Nursing Research* **21**:19–30

Ives, D G, Kuller, L H and Traven, N D (1993). Use and outcomes of a cholesterol-lowering intervention for rural elderly subjects. *American Journal of Preventive Medicine* **9**:274–81.

Kemper, D (1986). The healthwise program: growing younger. In: Dychtwald, K (ed.). *Wellness and Health Promotion for the Elderly.* Rockville, Maryland: Aspen Publishing.

Kirshner Associates, Inc. and Opinion Research Corporation (1983). *An evaluation of the nutrition services for the elderly*. Report submitted to administration on aging, DHHS, under contract 105-77-3002, Washington, DC.

Kupka Schutt, L and Mitchell, M E (1992). Positive effect of a nutrition instruction model on the dietary behavior of a selected group of elderly. *Journal of Nutrition for the Elderly* **12**(2):29– 53.

Lach, H W, Dwyer, J T and Mann, M (1994). P.E.P.: a partnership to assess and modify nutrition behavior in older adults. *Journal of Nutrition for the Elderly* **13**(3):57–67.

Lalonde, B, Hooyman, N and Blumhagen, J (1988). Long-term outcome effectiveness of a health promotion program for the elderly: the Wallingford Wellness Project. *Journal of Gerontological Social Work* **13**:95–112.

Lalonde, B I and FallCreek, S J (1985). Outcome effectiveness of the Wallingford Wellness Project: A model health promotion program for the elderly. *Journal of Gerontological Social Work* **9**(1):49–64.

Lave, J R, Ives, D G, Traven, N D and Kuller, L H (1996). Evaluation of a health promotion demonstration program for the rural elderly. *Health Services Research* **31**(3):261–81.

Lehmann, A B (1989). Under-nutrition in elderly people. *Age Ageing* **18**:339–53.

Leigh, J P, Richardson, N, Beck, R, Kerr, C, Harrington, H, Parcell, C L and Fries, J F (1992). Randomized controlled study of a retiree health promotion program: the Bank of America Study. *Archives of Internal Medicine* **152**(6):1201–6.

Lilley, J and Hunt, P (1998). *Opportunities for and barriers to change in the dietary behaviour of elderly people*. London: Health Education Authority.

Mayeda, C and Anderson, J (1993). Evaluating the effectiveness of the 'Self-CARE for a Healthy Heart' program with older adults. *Journal of Nutrition for the Elderly* **13**:11–22.

Mayer, J A, Jermanovich, A, Wright, B L, Elder, J P, Drew, J A and Williams, S J (1994). Changes in health behaviors of older adults: the San Diego Medicare Preventive Health Project. *Preventive Medicine* **23**(2):127–33.

Mitic, W (1985). Nutrition education for older adults: implementation of a nutrition instruction program. *Health Education* **16**(1):7–9.

Morrissey, J P, Harris, R P, Kincade Norburn, J, McLaughlin, C, Garrett, J M, Jackman, A M, Stein, J S, Lannon, C, Schwartz, R J and Patrick, D L (1995). Medicare reimbursement for preventive care: changes in performance of services, quality of life, and health care costs. *Medical Care* **33**(4):315–31.

Nelson, E C, McHugo, G, Schnurr, B A, Devito, C, Roberts, E, Simmons, J J and Zubkoff, W (1984). Medical self-care education for elders: a controlled trial to evaluate impact. *American Journal of Public Health* **74**(12):1357–62.

NHS Centre for Reviews and Dissemination (1996). *Undertaking systematic reviews of research on effectiveness: CRD guidelines for those carrying out or commissioning reviews*. CRD report No. 4. York: NHS CRD.

Office for National Statistics (1996). *National population projections 1994 based*. Series PP2 No. 20. London: Stationery Office.

Posner, B M, Jette, A M, Smith, K W and Miller, D R (1993). Nutrition and health risks in the elderly: the nutrition screening initiative [see comments]. *American Journal of Public Health* **83**(7):972–8.

Roe, L, Hunt, P, Bradshaw, H and Rayner, M (1997). *Review of the effectiveness of health promotion interventions to promote healthy eating*. London: Health Education Authority.

Rose, M A (1992). Evaluation of a peer-education program on heart disease prevention with older adults. *Public Health Nursing* **9**(4):242–7.

Schmidt, R M (1990). Evaluating outcomes of healthy ageing interventions: the HEALTH WATCH of Arizona Study in the Sun Cities. *Gerontologist* **30**:34A–36A.

Schweitzer, S O, Atchison, K A, Lubben, J E, Mayer Oakes, S A, De Jong, F J and Matthias, R E (1994). Health promotion and disease prevention for older adults: opportunity for change or preaching to the converted? *American Journal of Preventive Medicine* **10**(4):223–9.

Sehlub J, Jacques P F, Wilson P W F, Rush D and Rosenberg I H (1993). Vitamin status and intake as primary determinants of homocysteinemia in an elderly population. *JAMA* **270**:2693–8.

Simmons, J J, Nelson, E C, Roberts, E, Keller, A, Kane-Williams, E, Salisbury, Z T and Benson, L A (1989). Health Promotion Program: Staying Healthy after Fifty. *Health Education Quarterly* **16**:461–72.

Wechsler, R and Minkler, M (1986). A community-orientated approach to health promotion: the tenderloin senior outreach project. In: Dychtwald, K (ed.). *Wellness and Health Promotion for the Elderly*. Rockville: Aspen Publishing.

Weiss, E H and Davis, C H (1985). The response of an elderly audience to nutrition education articles in a newspaper for seniors. *Journal of Nutrition Education* **17**:197–202.

Winkleby, M A, Flora, J A and Kraemer, H C (1994). A community-based heart disease intervention: predictors of change. *American Journal of Public Health* **84**(5):767–72.